The Diggum Uppers

Body Snatching
and
Grave Robbing
in the
West Midlands

To Wendy

Kevin Goodman

The Diggum Uppers:
Body Snatching and Grave Robbing in the
West Midlands

Published by
Bows, Blades and Battles Press
202 Ashenhurst Road,
Dudley,
West Midlands,
Dy1 2hz.

ISBN 978-0-9571377-9-0

First published 2017 as
The Diggum Uppers:
Body Snatching and Grave Robbing in the Black
Country
This edition 2024

http://bowsbladesandbattles.tripod.com

Cover
Resurrectionists (1847), by Hablot Knight Browne.

For Amelia Caitlin Rose.

CONTENTS

ACKNOWLEDGMENTS

Many thanks to Luke Craddock–Bennett for a copy of his article *"Providence Chapel and burial ground, Sandwell, West Bromwich"* which set me off on an exploration of the activities of the resurrectionists in the West Midlands.

Picture Acknowledgements

Page 9: William Hunter. Stipple engraving by J. Thomson, 1847, after R. E. Pine. Wellcome Library, London.

Page 11: John Hunter. Line engraving by W. Sharp, 1788, after Sir J. Reynolds, 1786. Wellcome Library, London.

Page 12: Portrait of Sir Astley Paston Cooper, bust facing left. Stipple and line engraving 20th January 1824 by L. Alais. Wellcome Library, London.

Page 15: William Sands Cox by T.H. Maguire (1854). Wellcome Library, London.

Page 21: Dissection from Johannes Ketham *Fasiculo de medicina* (1491) Wellcome Library, London.

Page 22: Vesalius. *De humani corporis fabrica libri septem* ("On the fabric of the human body in seven books") (1543) Wellcome Library, London.

Page 25: William Hogarth *The dissection of the body of Tom Nero.* (1751) Wellcome Library, London.

Page 54: John Bishop, Thomas Williams, and James May: The Italian Boy Murderers) Wellcome Library, London.

Page 84: R.D. Grainger, Wellcome Library, London.

Page 96: Iron mort safe. Used with permission of the Science Museum.

The Diggum Uppers

Not A Trap Was Heard
(Anonymous Ballad c.1820)
Printed by Jackson & Son, Printers, 21, Moor-street, Birmingham.

NOT a trap was heard, or a Charley's note
As our course to the churchyard we hurried,
Not a pigman discharg'd a pistol shot
As a corpse from the grave we unburied.
We nibbled it slily at dead of night,
The sod with our pick-axes turning,
By the nosing moonbeam's chaffing light,
And our lanterns so queerly burning.
By the noosing, &c

Few and short were the words we said,
And we felt not a bit of sorrow,
But we rubb'd with rouge the face of the dead
And we thought of the spoil for to-morrow.
The useless shroud we tore from his breast
And then in regimentals bound him,
And he looked like a swaddy taking his rest,
With his lobster togs around him.
And he looked , &c

We thought as we fill'd up his narrow bed,
Our snatching trick now no look sees;
But the bulk and the sexton will find him fled,
And we far away towards Brooks's.
Largely they'll cheek 'bout the body that's gone
And poor Doctor Brooks they'll upbraid him;
But nothing we care if they leave him alone
In a place where a snatcher has laid him.
But nothing we care, &c

But half of our snatching job was o'er,
When a pal tipt the sign quick for shuffling,
And we heard by the distant hoarse Charley's roar
That the beaks would be 'mongst us soon scuffling.
Slily and slowly we laid him down,
In our cart famed for snatching in story;
Nicely and neatly we done 'em brown,
For we bolted away in our glory.
Nicely and neatly, &c

The Diggum Uppers

INTRODUCTION

The image frequently conjured of body snatchers or grave robbers: foggy, moonless nights in Edinburgh or London through which filthy, disheveled, rodent-featured men push wooden handcarts along cobbled back streets, the cargo not long dead or not long exhumed....

Such images are frequently coloured by the activities of William Burke and William Hare, the Scottish murderers who sold the bodies of their victims to the surgeon Dr Knox, or the London Italian Boy Murderers who operated around Shoreditch in London. The notion of it happening anywhere else, especially in the West Midlands, is rarely entertained. Yet in January 2013 archaeologists excavating the site of the former nineteenth century Providence Baptist Chapel and graveyard in Sandwell Road, West Bromwich, (founded 1810), discovered evidence of the attempts which were made to prevent corpses being stolen. One was an iron structure known as a *mortsafe*, designed to prevent the body being exhumed (Craddock-Bennett 2013). Other possible deterrents such as brick lined tombs have been discovered during excavations in St. Martin's Church yard and Park Street burial ground, Birmingham (Brickley at al 2006; Walker 2020).

Pushing the gothic speculations aside, this book examines the reasons for, and the reality behind, body snatching and grave robbing in the West Midlands. The first edition of this book, published in 2017, only covered the Black Country. This edition covers all the areas comprising the West Midlands (Herefordshire, Shropshire, Staffordshire, Warwickshire, and Worcestershire), and the once heavy industrial areas of Staffordshire and Worcestershire known as the Black Country[1], permitting even more interesting

---

[1] So called because of the filth and grime covering the surroundings; the product of the mining and iron-manufacturing industries which dominated the area.

stories to be told.

For example:

Birmingham:

RESURRECTIONISTS— This class of the profession appear to be again operating on our grave yards, with their usual daring and success. The body of Mr. Birch, late of Coleshill Street, of an advanced age, was abstracted from a grave to which it had the day before been consigned in the chapel yard of Ashted, one night last week, and carried off without detection.

On Sunday last, and aged couple, who the day before that followed the remains of their only offspring to the grave, visited the quiet retreat of Handsworth church yard, to cast another look upon the nearly raised turf, under which reposed the son who should have been the prop of their own declining years; when they found the grave disturbed and on further investigation, the sanctuary of the dead violated, the coffin broken, and the corpse carried away. This is the first instance of so brutal an outrage having been committed in this parish; and we hope from the activity of the church-wardens, that it may prove the last; indeed the precautions they have adopted to prevent a repetition of this misdemeanour, will most probably put a stop to it altogether. The reward of twenty pounds which has been offered, will be a greater temptation to those appointed to watch the living offenders, than any sum these miscreants may expect to raise by the sale of the dead[2].

Body Stolen. December 29, 1828. —Whereas, on Wednesday night, or early in the Morning of Christmas day, the Body of an aged Female was stolen from a Grave in Edgbaston Churchyard. A reward of Ten Pounds will be paid for such information as may lead

---

[2] p.2, *Birmingham Journal*, Saturday 18th October 1828.

to the conviction of the offenders, on application to the Churchwardens. (Langford 1871).

TWENTY GUINEAS REWARD.
WHEREAS late on Thursday night or early on Friday morning last, a CORPSE was stolen out of KING'S NORTON CHURCH-YARD: whoever will give such information as shall lead to the conviction of the offender or offenders shall receive TWENTY GUINEAS reward from the Churchwardens of the Parish.
And should the same offence be repeated, the above reward will be given to any one who shall give information that shall lead to the conviction of the offenders
November 10 1827.[3]

A few nights ago an attempt was made to raise the recently interred corpse of Mrs. Hopkins, from the church-yard of Yardley. It is supposed that these members of the profession were disturbed in their endeavours to obtain the body, as it was not taken away, although the earth had been entirely thrown out of the grave. At the desire of the friends of the deceased, the coffin was opened to ascertain the success of the miscreants. A parish meeting has been held for the purpose of adopting some measures to prevent any further attacks being made upon this cemetery.[4]

Coventry:

RESURRECTIONISTS IN COVENTRY.—On Wednesday, a considerable sensation was excited throughout this City, on it being discovered that some resurrectionists had been availing themselves of the facilities for disinterment, which are afforded by the exposed condition of the Church-yard.[5]

---

[3] p.2, *Aris's Birmingham Gazette*, Monday 12th November 1827.
[4] p.3, *Birmingham Journal*, Saturday 29th March 1828.
[5] p.3, *Birmingham Journal*, Saturday 11th July 1829.

To the EDITOR of the COVENTRY HERALD.

SIR. – Not doubting that a matter of such importance to all the neighbourhood will appear to you deserving of every publicity, I transmit the following for insertion in your next paper.

A CONSTANT READER.

In consequence of reports that resurrection men were in the neighbourhood, the attention of various individuals was attracted to the state of the recent graves in the church-yard of Manceter (which parish includes the township of Atherstone), and on Sunday last many persons remarked that one seemed very imperfectly filled, and that the soil lay scattered about, the sexton declaring that he believed that it had been disturbed, as it was in a state very different from that in which he had left it, and that he would examine it on the following morning. Accordingly, he did ascertain, by passing something down, that the coffin was there, but nothing farther. The friends, however, of the deceased, not satisfied with this, proceeded in the afternoon to clear out the grave, and were horror-struck at finding the body drawn out of the coffin to the loins, the head being raised almost to the surface, and left so. Probably the process of decay had been so rapid as to make it useless as a subject; the internment had taken place on the preceding Monday, and the attempt is supposed to have been made on the following Wednesday night, as a stranger person of suspicious appearance was observed to come up on that day from towards Atherstone, and loiter about examining the church-yard and the avenues to it, It is said that a sum of sixteen guineas was offered for the corpse, and refused; a circumstance which, if true, may reasonably point suspicion at the instigators of this revolting practice of violating the sanctuary of the dead. It is reported that other cemeteries in the neighbourhood have also been visited.[6]

---

[6] p.3, *Coventry Herald*, Friday, 18th February 1825.

RESURRECTIONS AT STONELEIGH.

A gentleman residing in Stoneleigh, a village five miles distant from Coventry, having noticed two suspicious-looking fellows about the Parish Church-yard, on Sunday last, it occurred to him that they were resurrectionists, reconnoitering with a view to a snatch. He accordingly, on that night, ordered two of his men to go to the Church-yard, and remain there concealed for some time; they did so, and between twelve and one o'clock, two men entered the burial-ground, proceeded to the grave in which Mr. John Newbold (who committed suicide last week,) was interred and commenced removing the soil with implements which they brought with them; at this moment the sentinels, over anxious for the capture of these nightly depredators, started forth towards the grave, but the resurrectionists seeing them, made off, and effected their escape.[7]

BODY-SNATCHING.– Considerable alarm has been excited among the inhabitants of Allesley, within the last few days, in consequence of some resurrection-men practising their unhallowed and disgusting vocation in the church-yard of that village. On the morning of yesterday week (Thursday), as a person was going to ring the six o'clock bell, he discovered, on entering the church-yard, that the grave of Joseph Arnett, an old man, aged 70, who was buried about seven weeks since, had been disturbed; he went immediately and gave an alarm, when, on opening the grave, they found the body taken away. Suspicion fell upon two strange men who had been drinking at the Rainbow public-house, the previous afternoon, and who had had a large box made which they said was intended for a tool-chest; however, neither the men, the box, nor the body were to be found, and the alarm subsided till Saturday evening, when some boards, cut to the size of a large box, but not nailed together, were found under a hedge by the road side near Allesley.

---

[7] p.4, *Coventry Herald,* Friday 16th April 1830

Supposing the depredators were about to pay another visit, ten of the villagers sat up all night to watch the church-yard, as they had done on the Thursday evening, and two were p laced so as to see if any one came for the boards, but all remained quiet. On Sunday, Mr. Hollick, the headborough, conceiving there might be some snatching implement hid near, searched the hedges and ditches of the fields in the neighbourhood, when, during the time of service in the afternoon, he found a sack containing a human body, in a gorse bush, near a pit, belonging to Mr. Hayward, about a quarter of a mile from Allesley, on the Birmingham road; two persons were placed to watch during the night, but no one came and on Monday morning the sack was taken to the White Lion, when the body was identified as that of Joseph Arnett, and in the course of the day it was re-committed to its troubled habitation in the church-yard.[8]

BODY STEALING – On Saturday, as a man was gathering elderberries in Budbrook Church-yard, [Warwickshire] *near this town, he perceived that one of the graves had lately been disturbed. On communicating this circumstance to some of the neighbours, who went back with him, they suspected, from finding a piece of coffin lying in the grass and the disordered state of the top of a grave in which the remains of a poor woman of the name of Ann Yarne had lately been interred, that the body had been stolen. On Sunday morning, a chisel, and a long stick, which had been used, as it is supposed, in trying the depth of the grave, were found near the place; and the son of the deceased, having obtained leave, had the grave opened, when it was ascertained that the body had been extracted. On opening the grave, several pieces of skin and flesh were found among the earth. The deceased was about 80 years of*

---

[8] p.4, *Coventry Herald*, Friday 5th March 1830

age. It is thought that the body had been stolen on Friday night.[9]

Worcester:

Resurrection Men. – These disturbers of the dead have made their appearance in Worcester; they stole on Tuesday eight last, from St. Andrew's church-yard, the body of a female which was interred on Monday.[10]

APPREHENSION OF A GANG OF RESURRECTION MEN. – On Saturday night last, four men were taken up at Worcester, in whose possession eight dead bodies were found, viz. three men, two women, and three children. The bodies are supposed to have been stolen in that neighbourhood.[11]

---

[9] p.4, *Coventry Herald*, Friday 8th October 1830.
[10] p.3, *Staffordshire Advertiser*, Saturday 15th October 1814.
[11] p.4, *Coventry Herald*, Friday 8th February 1828.

1.MEDICAL DEMAND

It could be argued that the Body Snatchers and Grave robbers, or to give them any of their other titles: *"Resurrection Men"*, *"Resurrectionists"*, *"Snatchers"*, *"Grabs"*, *"Lifters"*, *"Body Stealers"*, *"Body Lifters"*, *"Exhumaters"*, *"Diggum Uppers"* *"Sack 'em up men"*, or *"Resurgem Homo"*, supplying the anatomy schools and medics of the past, are a distasteful episode in the annals of medical history, (from hereon, for simplicity, they will be referred to as *"Resurrectionists"*)[12].

However, it cannot be denied it is an episode that has captured the public imagination; with many books (both fiction and non-fiction), documentaries, films, websites and tours around Edinburgh and London devoted to them.

Dissection of human cadavers (dead bodies) is recognized as necessary in the training of physicians and surgeons, and to advance medical science. Today, it is governed by strict ethical guidelines (Bhattarai et al 2022): the Human Tissue Act (2004) in England, Wales, and Northern Ireland; the Human Tissue Act (2006) in Scotland, and the Human Tissue Authority. The Human Tissue Authority is an independent regulator of organisations that remove, store, and use human tissue for research, medical treatment, post-mortem examination, education, and training[13].

Many influential physicians and surgeons, who have made major contributions to the advancement of medical science have been the patrons of resurrectionists. For example:

William Hunter (1718-1783): Scottish anatomist, physician and obstetrician and physician to Queen Charlotte (1744-1818), wife of

---

[12] The term "Burkers" is not included as it is derived from "Burking": a method of killing by suffocation used by William Burke, the murderer and resurrectionists, hence its title.

[13] https://www.hta.gov.uk

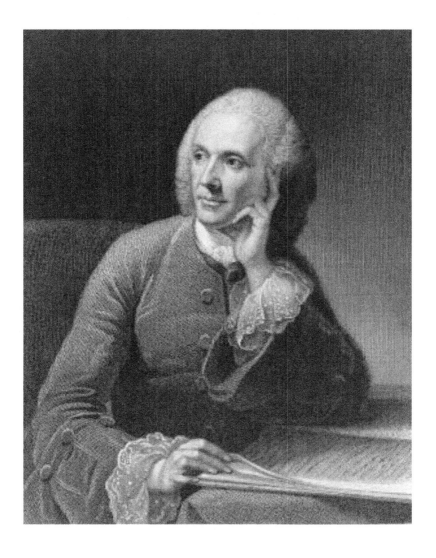

William Hunter (1718-1783) (Wellcome Images)

King George III (1738-1820). While famous for his studies on bone and cartilage, his greatest work was *"Anatomia uteri humani gravidi," ("On the anatomical details of uterus and fetus at different stages")* (1774). He founded the Hunterian Medical school at his home on Great Windmill Street, Soho, London in 1768. (Ghosh and Kumar 2021).

John Hunter (1728-1793): William's brother. A surgeon, teacher and anatomist, and surgeon to King George III. He helped to improve understanding of human teeth; bone growth; inflammation; gunshot wounds; venereal diseases; digestion; child development; the separateness of maternal and fœtal blood supplies, and the role of the lymphatic system. He opened his first anatomy school in Piccadilly, London, in 1764, and a larger one at his home in Leicester Square in 1783 (Moore 2006).

Sir Astley Paston Cooper (1768-1841): Contributed to the understanding of ontology, vascular surgery, anatomy and pathology of the mammary glands and testicles, and the pathology and surgery of hernias. He taught at St Thomas's Hospital, London (Burch 2007).

The resurrectionists' leading patron in the West Midlands was William Sands Cox (1802-1875), one of the founders of Birmingham Medical School in Temple Row, Birmingham.

Early training of surgeons was through apprenticeships usually lasting seven years - physicians were university trained. During this time, the apprentice, along with several others, would be taught by his master, assisting him during procedures and attending classes at anatomy schools. Eventually the apprentice took an examination; after 1745, this was conducted by the Surgeons' Company and after 1800 by The Royal College of Surgeons. If successful they were awarded a diploma and permitted to practice (Porter 1998).

The first public medical teaching in Birmingham was delivered by John Tomlinson, the first surgeon to the Birmingham Workhouse

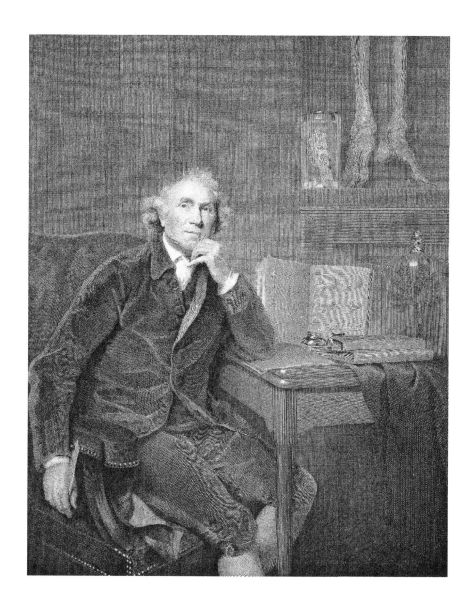

John Hunter (1728-1793) (Wellcome Images)

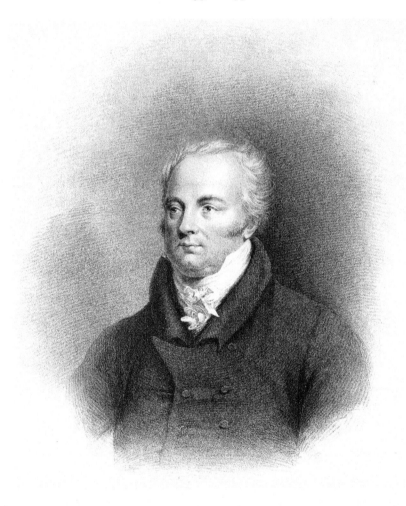

Sir Astley Paston Cooper (1768-1841)
(Wellcome Images)

Infirmary, and later to Birmingham General Hospital. Tomlinson delivered a course of twenty-eight weekly lectures on anatomy during 1767-1768 at the Birmingham Workhouse, probably utilizing the cadavers of those who had died there. These classes were among the earliest formal medical lectures to be held outside Scotland and London, traditional centres of medical education. Lectures involving anatomical dissection usually took place from October to May, the coolest months (Reinarz 2009).

Advertisements for Anatomical lectures appeared in *Aris' Birmingham Gazette* in 1768. They were to be held in the Great Room at Cooke's Coffee House, in the Cherry Orchard, in the area between Temple Row and High Street. Although it is unknown who delivered them:

BIRMINGHAM, OCT. 24, 1768.
IN COOKE'S Great-Room, in the Cherry-Orchard, on Thursday next, at Five of the Clock in the Afternoon, will be given an INTRODUCTORY LECTURE, previous to a COURSE of ANATOMICAL LECTURES, which will be continued Weekly, (or oftener when proper Subjects occur) till the whole Course is completed.
    The Design is to demonstrate in a plain and concise Method, the Structure of the Human Body, under the following Divisions:

1 *OSTEOLOGY*, [skeleton and bones]
2 *SARCOLOGY*, [the soft parts.]
3 *NEUROLOGY* [nervous system]
4 *SPLANCHRONOLOGY*, [the visceral organs]
5 *MYOLOGY*, [muscles]
6 *ANGIOLOGY*, [circulatory system]
7 *ADENOLOGY* [glands.]

More Particulars will be explained in the Introductory Lecture. Tickets for Admittance to be had at Pearson and Aris's Printers.

BIRMINGHAM, Nov. 7, 1768.

IN COOKE'S Great-Room, in the Cherry-Orchard, this Afternoon, at Five o' Clock, will begin An Anatomical Lecture EXTRAORDINARY, On the fresh Human Fœtus, with the Arteries injected. In this Lecture will be exhibited a general View of the most considerable Organs in the Body, and the Particularities of the Fœtus will be described. On every Wednesday, at Four o'Clock in the Afternoon, the Course of Lectures will be continued as first proposed. The Terms to Subscribers are One Guinea for the whole Course, to Non-Subscribers Two Shillings each Lecture.

No doubt *"when proper Subjects occur"* is a synonym for the availability of cadavers.

Cox was the eldest son of the Birmingham surgeon Edward Townsend Cox (1769-1863), surgeon to the Birmingham workhouse (founded 1734). Educated at Birmingham's King Edward VI Grammar School, he began his medical training under the supervision of his father and later studied medicine at Birmingham General Hospital (founded 1779). From 1821 to 1823, he studied at Guy's and St Thomas' Hospitals, London, and was admitted as a Member of the Royal College of Surgeons (MRCS). In 1824, he continued his education at the École de Médecine, Paris, returning to Birmingham in 1825, and becoming surgeon at the General Dispensary[14].

He advertised a series of lectures on '*Anatomical*

---

[14] Dispensaries were charitable institutions which provided free medical advice and treatment to the sick poor. They were first established in the seventeenth century in Edinburgh (1682) and London (c1690), by 1800 around 40 were in operation around the country (Whitfield 2016). To William Hutton their purpose was *"To supply the industrious of the labouring classes, who are not able to pay a surgeon for his services, with medical and surgical relief, for the payment of a trifling subscription. It also affords, by the contribution of the opulent and benevolent, relief to those who are unable to contribute any sum themselves"* (Lane 2001)

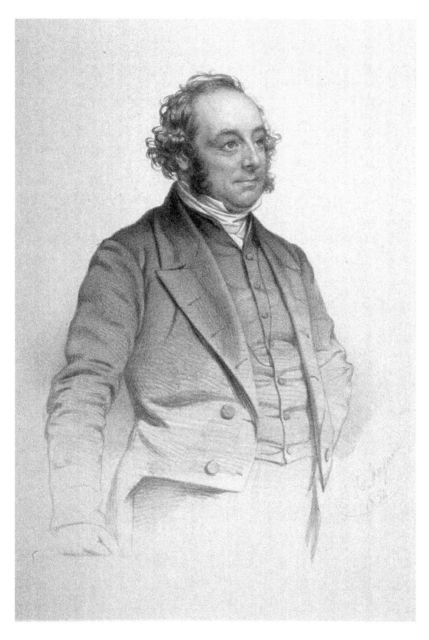

William Sands Cox by T.H. Maquire (1854)
(Wellcome Images)

MR. W. S. COX will commence a course of ANATOMICAL DEMONSTRATIONS, with Surgical and Physiological Observations, on Wednesday the 1st of December, at twelve o'clock, and which will be continued during the ensuing winter on Mondays, Wednesdays, and Fridays, at 24, Temple-row.—W. S. C. has great gratification in stating that the plan he proposes to pursue has met with the decided approbation and sanction of Dr. Johnstone, Dr. Pearson, the Physicians and Surgeons of the Hospital, Dispensary, Town Infirmary, and other distinguished Practitioners.

For particulars and prospectus of the course apply at 24, Temple-row.

Advertisement for William Sands Cox's Anatomy lectures.
(*Aris' Birmingham Gazette,* 7th November 1825)
(Author's Collection)

September 23, 1823.

BIRMINGHAM

SCHOOL OF MEDICINE AND SURGERY.

PATRONS.

MARQUESS of LANSDOWNE   The LORD BISHOP of the
EARL FITZWILLIAM   DIOCESE
EARL SPENCER   The Hon. Mr. LYTTELTON
EARL PLYMOUTH   Sir GREY SKIPWITH, Bart.
EARL of BRADFORD   Sir ROBERT PEEL, Bart.
EARL HOWE   Sir J. E. E. WILMOT, Bart.
EARL MOUNTNORRIS   D. S. DUGDALE, Esq. M.P.
Lord Viscount HOOD   F. LAWLEY, Esq. M.P.

WINTER SESSION.

THIS COURSE of LECTURES will commence on Monday, November the 3d.

An Introductory Discourse will be delivered by Dr. PEARSON, at the Rooms of the Lecturers, at the Birmingham Institution, in Temple-row, on that day, at one o'clock.

ANATOMY, PHYSIOLOGY, and PATHOLOGY, with Dissections and Examinations, by Mr. W. S. Cox—Mondays, Wednesdays, Fridays, and Saturdays, at one o'clock.

MATERIA MEDICA and MEDICAL BOTANY, by Dr. PEARSON and Dr. ECCLES—Tuesdays and Fridays, at one o'clock.

CHEMISTRY and PHARMACY, by Mr. WOOLRICH—Mondays and Thursdays, at seven o'clock in the evening.

The *SPRING SESSION* will commence in the first week of February next.

The Introductory Lecture will be delivered by Dr. BOOTH.

PRINCIPLES and PRACTICE of PHYSIC, with practical Instructions and Examinations, by Dr. BOOTH—Mondays and Thursdays, at one o'clock.

PRINCIPLES and PRACTICE of SURGERY, with practical Instructions and Examinations, by Mr. JUKES—Tuesdays and Fridays, at seven o'clock in the evening.

PRINCIPLES and PRACTICE of MIDWIFERY, with Cases, by Mr. INGLEBY—Wednesdays and Saturdays, at seven o'clock in the evening.

For Terms and other particulars application may be made to the Lecturers respectively, or to Mr. W. S. Cox, Honorary Secretary, 24, Temple-row.

Advertisement for the Birmingham School of Medicine and Surgery
(Author's collection)

Demonstrations with Surgical and Physiological Observations for students in *Aris' Birmingham Gazette* (7th November 1825) (see page 16), commencing on December 1st, 1825, at his father's house at 24 Temple Row, nineteen people enrolled. These lectures involved the dissection of cadavers, which Reinarz (2009) speculates *"... access to which was certainly facilitated by the work that Edward Cox undertook as one of the surgeons to the workhouse infirmary."* (p.47). Their popularity and the rapidly increasing number of students encouraged Sands Cox to abandon teaching in his father's house and seek larger premises.

In 1828, in conjunction with several medical men, including Doctors Edward Johnstone and John Kaye Booth, physicians to the General Hospital, he founded the Birmingham School of Medicine and Surgery, comprising a lecture theatre, dissecting room, library, and anatomy museum at Snow Hill. The expansion of the school resulted in a move to Paradise Street in 1834. King William IV accepted the office of Patron of the school in 1836 and the medical school became known as *"The Birmingham Royal School of Medicine and Surgery"*. In October 1841 on Bath Row, Sands Cox and his colleagues founded the Queen's Hospital as a teaching hospital supporting the medical school. It was one of the first hospitals opened specifically as a teaching hospital - staff were appointed on the understanding they had to give instruction to students. Queens was granted a Royal Charter by Queen Victoria in 1843 establishing it as Queen's College (Morrison 1926).

Dissection.

The dissection of human cadavers was first practiced by the Greek physicians Herophilos (c330-c260 B.C.) and Erasistratos (c310-c250 B.C.) at the School of Anatomy in Alexandria. Forbidden in the Roman world, the physician and surgeon Galen of Pergamon (129AD-200 AD) was forced to dissect Barbary apes and pigs.

Unfortunately, based on his findings, which he generalized to humans, he made several errors regarding the heart and circulation, and reproductive organs. These errors persisted through the centuries (Nutton 2004), his conclusions remaining uncontested until the sixteenth century when the anatomist Andreas Vesalius (1514-1564) published *his De humani corporis fabrica libri septem* ("*On the Fabric of The Human Body in Seven Books*") in 1543 (O'Malley 1964).

In the early Christian and Islamic worlds, the practice of cadaver dissection was forbidden. In 1231, the Holy Roman Emperor Frederick II (1194-1250) decreed that a human dissection should be performed at the *Schola Medica Salernitana*, the Medical School at Salerno, Italy, at least once every five years. It was legalized in various parts of the Holy Roman Empire and was introduced into the study of anatomy at the University of Bologna, Italy, around 1300. It was in Bologna that Mondino de Liuizzi (1275-1326) performed the first public display of dissection in 1315. During the fourteenth century, the Universities of Perugia, Padua, and Florence made it mandatory for candidates for the doctorate degree in medicine to attend at least one dissection. In 1387, the Statutes of the University of Florence requested the authorities to deliver the bodies of three foreign executed prisoners annually for dissection, establishing the connection between punishment and dissection (Goodman 1944; Quigley 2012; Rengachary et al 2009). In the British Isles, permission was granted on July 1st, 1505, by the Town Council of Edinburgh in the "*Seal of Cause to the Barbers and Surgeons of Edinburgh*" (ratified by King James IV of Scotland the following year):

We may have anis in the year, ane condampnit man efter he be deid to make anatomea of quhairthrow we mayhaif experience Ilk ane to instruct uthers And we sail do suffrage for the soule. [We may have once a year a condemned man after he be dead, to make anatomy of, wherethrough we may have experience to instruct others. And we shall do suffrage for the soul.] (p49-50, Lonsdale 1870)

The surgeons of England and Wales were granted the right to dissect in 1540 in the Charter given by King Henry VIII to the United Company of Barbers and Surgeons:

... the sayd maysters or governours of the mistery and comminaltie of barbours and surgeons of London, and their successours yerely for ever after their said discrecions at their free liberte and pleasure shal and maie have and take without contradiction foure persons condempned adiudged and put to death for feloni by the due order of the Kynges lawe of thys realme for anatomies without any further sute or labour to be made to the kynges highnes his heyres or successours for the same. And to make incision of the same deade bodies or otherwyse to order the same after their said discrecions at their pleasure for their further and better knowlage instruction insight learning and experience in the sayd scyence or facultie or surgery (p.588, Young 1890).

During the Renaissance, medics were not the only profession performing dissections. Artists also performed them. The Florentine painter Antonio Pollainolo (1431/1432-1498) dissected many human bodies to investigate the muscles and understand the human body. Leonardo da Vinci (1452-1519), Michelangelo Buanorotti (1475-1564), and Baccio Bandinelli (1493-1560), all conducted anatomical dissections, enabling them to set new standards in their depictions of the human body (Sellmer 2001).

In 1565, Elizabeth I granted the Royal College of Physicians four cadavers annually for dissection, and Charles II increased Henry's original grant to the Barbers and Surgeons to six in 1663 (Quigley 2012).

In 1694, the grant made by the Town Council of Edinburgh was extended for the medical schools to include:

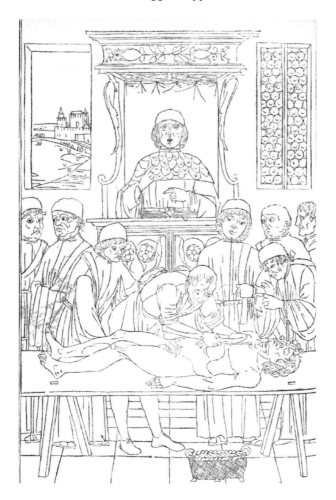

Dissection
Johannes de Ketham, *Fasiculo de medicina* (1491)
(Wellcome Images)

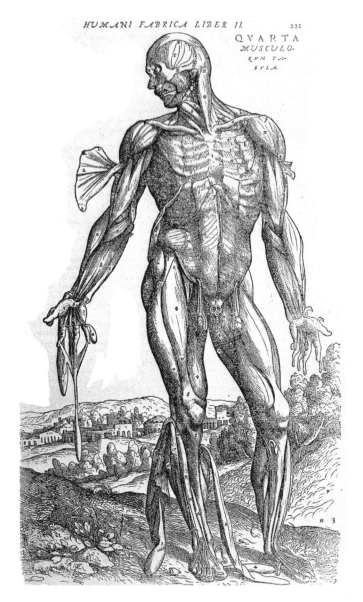

Vesalius.
De humani corporis fabrica libri septem (1543)
("*On The Fabric of The Human Body in Seven Books*")
(Wellcome Images)

... those bodies that dye in the correction-house; the bodies of fundlings who dye betwixt the tyme that they are weaned and thir being put to schools or trades; also the dead bodies of such that are stifiet in the birth, which are exposed, and have none to owne them; as also the dead bodies of such as are felo de se [suicide]*; likewayes the bodies of such as are put to death by sentence of the magistrat"* (p807, Goodman 1944).

By the eighteenth century the power of the monopolies of the Company of Barber-Surgeons and the Royal College of Physicians was waning, the Company of Barber-Surgeons would cease in 1745 when the surgeons split to form the Company of Surgeons. In 1800, the Company was granted a royal charter to become the Royal College of Surgeons in London, and in 1843 it became the Royal College of Surgeons of England (Bolwell 2022). The great London hospitals of St. Thomas and St. Bartholomew were teaching anatomy, and private schools run by former hospital lecturers, such as the Hunter brothers, soon appeared. The demand for anatomical subjects was growing. As part of the 1751 Murder Act under George II, common law provision was made for the statutory dissection of murderers:

It is thereby become necessary, that some further terror and peculiar mark of infamy be added to the punishment of death, now by law inflicted on such as shall be guilty of the said heinous offence ... which sentence shall be expressed not only the usual judgment of death, but also the time appointed hereby for the execution thereof, and the marks of infamy hereby directed for such offenders, in order to impress a just horror in the mind of the offender, and on the, minds of such as shall be present, of the heinous crime of murder.[15]

---

[15] https://statutes.org.uk/site/the-statutes/eighteenth-century/1751-25-geo2-c37-murder-act/

Dissection was used as a punishment as it was regarded as a desecration of the dead, and it was feared it would prevent a spirit's resurrection on Judgement Day (Bennett 2017).

West Midland murderers who were dissected following execution include: Joseph Darby of Featherless Barn, Halesowen, who In April 1759, together with his two sons, murdered a local bailiff, John Walker. Darby and his sons were found guilty and hanged at Shrewsbury Assizes, Darby's body was given to the surgeons for dissection and his sons' bodies were hung in chains, in Gibbet Lane, (today Alexander Road), Halesowen (see Appendix 1). Abel Hill drowned his common law wife Mary Martin and their two-year-old son, Thomas, in a Bilston canal in February 1820. He was hanged on 27th July at Stafford and his body publicly dissected by the surgeon Edward Best at Workhouse Fold, Bilston (see Appendix 2)[16]. Hill's skeleton was preserved by Dr. Tom Dickenson of Bilston High Street who had a macabre sense of humour, according to Freeman (1931):

The doctor had a way of his own, and had the bones wired in their places, and the complete skeleton fixed in an upright position in a specially constructed cabinet. The turn of a knob caused the doors to open, and the uncanny thing to stretch out its bony arms. From Dr. Dickenson the grim relic passed to Dr. Best, in whose surgery it remained for some years, until one dark night when it was taken out, and secretly buried." (p12)

In 1830, Charles Wall of Oldswinford was hanged at Worcester Prison for the murder of his fiancée's daughter, Sally. He was dissected at Worcester's Infirmary Hospital (Appendix 3).

By 1760, it had become customary in the anatomical schools

---

[16] Freeman (1931) claimed Hill's ghost was subsequently seen in the locale.

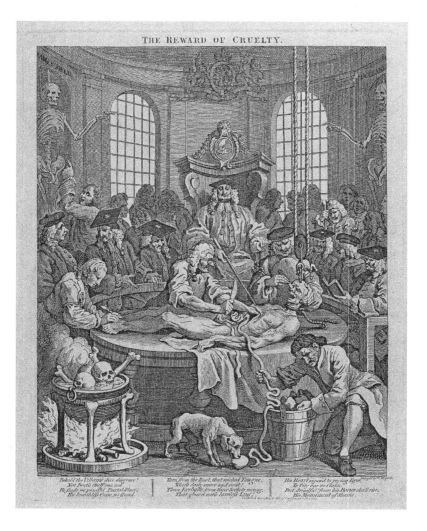

William Hogarth (1697-1764)
The dissection of the body of Tom Nero. (1751)
(Wellcome Images)

for students to dissect for themselves. It was also mandatory for those applying for licenses from the Royal College of Surgeons to attend two full courses in anatomy with dissection. Practicing surgeons also liked to operate at least once on a cadaver before performing a difficult operation (Hurren 2011; Wise 2004).

The demand for anatomical material escalated.

In Edinburgh, the number of medical students in Edinburgh was fifty-seven in 1720; approximately three hundred and forty in 1780-90, and over four hundred after 1800. In London in 1793, there were over two hundred medical students and over a thousand by 1823. Each student required three bodies during his sixteen months of training: two for learning anatomy and one on which to practice operating techniques. Sir Astley Cooper estimated that in 1828 about four hundred and fifty cadavers were dissected in the London schools in one season (Goodman 1944; Hurren 2011; Wise 2004).

The supply of convicted murderers was insufficient. The surgeons and the students were competing for less than a hundred cadavers legally available each year. And the number was diminishing - in 1805, sixty-eight people were executed in England and Wales, by 1831 this had dropped to fifty-two as the punishment of deportation became more common (Hurren 2011; Wise 2004).

It was a market ready to be exploited.

2. THE RISE OF THE RESURRECTIONISTS

At first, the grave-robbers were amateurs, usually medical students or hospital porters who stole for their own use or their surgeons. Morrison (1926) notes:

An esteemed local doctor narrates the exploits of his grandfather when a medical student about 1820 to Mr. Saunders, a practitioner in Islington Row; the master and pupil obtaining a body from Edgbaston Churchyard, and bringing it away wrapped in a long coat and propped up on the seat of the gig between the two accomplices. (p.19)

Although this ploy could backfire:

The Dead Alive —The resurrection men have adopted a new plan to prevent detection, by dressing the bodies which they steal, so that if seen they appear asleep. A few days ago two of them, coming from the country, stopped at a public-house, about four miles from town, with the body of a man, whom, after violating the grave, they dressed in the uniform of a soldier. While in the house, taking refreshment, a soldier who was billeted there, went to the door to smoke his pipe, and curiosity having induced him to look into the cart, he perceived a soldier, as he supposed asleep, whom in the first instance he conceived to be a deserter, and hailed him with "Halloo, comrade, where to?" not receiving an answer, he attempted to awake the corpse, exclaiming, "Come, my boy, let us have something to drink." No answer being made , he went to the ostler, and they examined the body, when the latter expressed his suspicion that the fellows, who were in the house, "were Body-snatchers," and he and the soldier held a council of war, as to what steps they should pursue, when it was agreed to convey the dead man into the stable, and that the soldier should occupy his place in the cart, while the ostler would follow on horse-back to assist him in case of need. This was accordingly done, and the Snatchers having refreshed, drove off with the cart, but they had not proceeded a hundred yards before they found the supposed dead man tumble about, and stopped to remedy the inconvenience. On taking hold of him, one of the fellows observed. "Ise be cursed if this here subject is'nt warm" – the other having felt him, said, "Dam un, but he's hot;" – "and so would you, too," said the soldier, "if you had come from h_ll, where I have been." This was enough; the snatchers were petrified, and almost terrified to death; but as soon as they recovered they set off, leaving the cart and horse in possession of the soldier and ostler, neither of which has since been owned. The body of the dead man was in two days after restored to his friends, by whom it was missed from the grave[17].

Langley (1978) relates a variant of the above tale in which the soldier is replaced by the Black Country bare knuckle fighter, William Perry, "The Tipton Slasher" (1819–1880), and the incident takes place just outside Wolverhampton, claiming the tale was told to him by his *"great aunt who was born in 1848"* (p.7).

While stationed in Kidderminster as an assistant surgeon with the Royal Lancashire Regiment as part of his military service, Joseph Jordan (1787 –1873), (later to establish a medical school in Manchester, and become a Fellow of the Royal College of Surgeons), engaged in grave robbing. He was *"… pounced upon by an outraged father and mother for being in possession of the corpse of their child."* (p.23, Jordan 1904), as a result he was forced to leave Kidderminster swiftly (Jordan 1904).

With the increase in demand for cadavers, the resurrectionists soon became organised. At first, they were mostly cemetery watchmen, aided by a few individuals. By the early nineteenth century several well-organised gangs of resurrectionists had appeared in London and other large cities, including Birmingham.

---

[17] p.2, *Hereford Journal*, Wednesday 2nd April 1823.

Over a period of fifteen months during 1830-1832, seven gangs were arrested in London. At that time, the London resurrectionists were estimated to number approximately two hundred. Some of the most effective resurrectionists were able to exhume, discreetly, about ten bodies during a single night (Wise 2004).

The operations of a Birmingham gang were revealed when a cadaver in a packing case was discovered at a Birmingham coach office:

BIRMINGHAM RESURRECTIONISTS. – On Thursday last, in consequence of informations received at the Public Office, Palmer the officer, went to Bird's coach office, in Constitution-hill where a box was given into his custody, directed to "J.Blythe, Esq. Black Bull Inn, Edinburgh." On opening the package, it proved to contain the body of a female, about 50 years of age, which had apparently, from incisions in the abdomen, undergone a surgical postmortem examination. The Clerk at the office, who, upon suspecting what was contained in the box was the first to communicate his suspicions to the police, states that the package was brought by two men, whom he should again know. They had before brought similar packages, but he never suspected their contents. On the 15th of October, the same men took to the office a similar box, directed to a "Mr. Thompson, Edinburgh;" and on the 11th of November, another to the same gentleman; on the 29th of November, one to Mr. Blandford of London; on the 1st December, one to Mr. Blythe of Edinburgh; and on the 13th inst. Another for the same individual. The latter has been intercepted, and we are not without hopes, that the discovery will lead to the detection of an infamous gang, who are notorious for having carried on the trade in dead bodies to a very considerable extent in this town and neighbourhood. The box after coming into the possession of the Police was taken to the prison in Moor-street, and from thence yesterday morning removed to the work-house to await the verdict of a coroner's inquest[18]

The recipients may have been agents working for the anatomy schools or individual surgeons.

According to Palmer (2007) and an article entitled *"Black Country Body Snatchers"* in the *Black Country Bugle* (June 18th, 2014) by Josephine Jasper, a man named *"Brummajem Booth"* who lived in Rowley, led a gang of resurrectionists who operated throughout the Black Country, transporting the bodies to the Birmingham medical school in farm carts concealed under straw and other merchandise.

Palmer also includes the following (unsourced) rhyme:

Here in 1825,
A mon's wuth mower jed than alive
If yow dow believe this dyin' truth
Have a word with Brummagem Booth

Unfortunately, both Mr. Palmer and Ms. Jasper fail to provide the source for their information, so, at best, their accounts must be regarded as local lore.

The *Staffordshire Advertiser* (Saturday, 21st March 1829) reported a group of resurrectionists attempting to solicit business from Stafford doctors and surgeons:

A "professional" person, in the "Resurrection" line, with two assistants, has been lingering about this town several days during the week. He applied to our medical practitioners; but, in consequence of their being too busy with patients to attend to "subjects," he did not obtain a single order. If any violation of the grave had been attempted, police officers were prepared to seize the perpetrators. The fellows are believed now to have left the town; and for the information of neighbouring constables, we are requested to

---

[18] p.2, *Birmingham Journal*, Saturday 17th December 1831.

state that the head man is nearly six feet high, about 45 years of age, has a scarred face, large whiskers trained down to his chin, wears a drab great coat, drab hat, and top boots, and has a confidant bullying demeanour. (p.4)

Resurrection gangs had no hesitation in invading other gangs' territories, including Birmingham:

...a gang of resurrection men have recently visited this neighbourhood from London, intending to furnish "subjects" for the winter lectures from the church-yards in this town. An attempt was made this week to remove a corpse that had been interred in St. Martin's church-yard, and every night since a watch has been set upon the grave. We understand that finding their attempts in the town were hazardous, they have laid their scene of action at a few miles distance, though still hovering round Birmingham, as the centre of their attraction[19]

And in Ashted, Birmingham:

A RESURRECTION MAN APPREHENDED. On Friday morning last the constable of the night, on returning from his rounds by Ashted Chapel, perceived two men carrying between them a large bag, covered with green cloth. This circumstance aroused his suspicions; when on being joined by a watchman, he hastened in pursuit of the men, and was on the point of overtaking them, when the gentlemen finding their escape becoming hopeless, threw down their burden and took to their heels. The pursuit now become hot, and terminated at length in one of the pursued becoming a prisoner; the other unfortunately made his escape and has not since been heard of. On examining the bag, it was found to contain a dead body! Which afterwards was proved to be that of a man named George Ireland, who died a short time since, and was interred in

---

[19] p.2, *Birmingham Journal*, Saturday, 17th November 1827.

Ashted Chapel-yard. The man who was secured was shortly after lodged in the prison, and on Monday last was brought up, and underwent a long examination at our Public Office. He states his name to be Thomas Thompson, and says he is a native of Cropthorne, near Croydon, Surrey, but refuses to give any information of his companion. He was remanded and will be again brought up before the Magistrates this day. The body which was disinterred has been again committed to the earth, in the presence of the afflicted relatives and friends of the deceased.[20]

We are informed that resurrection men, as they are called are going up and down the country, and that two of these fellows stopped at Stone, a few days ago, with full attention of executing their purpose, but the officers of the place having discovered their design, immediately took one of them into custody, and he has been committed as a vagrant to Stafford Gaol, for a month's hard labour. – The other man escaped, but information having been given of his route, we hope he will be apprehended.[21]

Despite the risk of imprisonment if caught, the financial rewards of grave robbing were great. A weekly wage for a factory worker in the first quarter of the nineteenth century was approximately 7 shillings; for a skilled tailor or carpenter: 30 shillings, and for a well-paid manservant in a wealthy household: 1 guinea a week. A cadaver, depending upon freshness and demand, could fetch between 8-20 guineas (Hurren 2011). In March 1812, the London Borough Gang stole 44 adult cadavers and 7 smalls (children) (Bailey 1896) - a considerable sum when sold.

Some cadavers commanded a high premium. Male cadavers were more sought after than female ones, due to their musculature. Fresh cadavers and limbs commanded a higher price than ones on

---

[20] p.7, *Birmingham Chronicle*, Thursday 5th May 1825
[21] P.4, *Staffordshire Advertiser*, Saturday 12th June 1824

the verge of putrefaction. Children's bodies (known as "*smalls*") commanded a high price as did specialty cadavers: those with congenital disorders or illnesses or had died in an unusual manner (Wise 2004). For example, the surgeon John Hunter paid £500 to procure the body of the Irish giant Charles O'Byrne (1761-1783), whose eight-foot skeleton Hunter wanted for his anatomical museum. This may have been the reason the person buried at the Providence Baptist Chapel in West Bromwich was interred in a mort safe: it belonged to a young woman (aged 17-25), who in life had suffered from a disfiguring skin and bone disease, possibly metastatic cancer[22]: her body would have fetched a high premium for a resurrectionist (Craddock-Bennett. 2013). A person dying of a sporting injury would also be profitable:

Death by Fighting.— A sanguinary fight took place at Erdington, near Birmingham, on Monday, which terminated in the death of one of the combatants. The principals were William Fitter, a working and Thomas Hill, a thimble maker. The match, which led to the fatal fight, was made for a sovereign aside; and the place chosen for the fight was a field adjoining to the Horse-shoe public-house, at Gravelly-hill. On Monday the combatants met, Fitter being seconded by two men, named Barton and fight was one of the most determined ever witnessed; and at the termination of the 48th round Fitter was taken up lifeless, and his antagonist afterwards carried home in a most dangerous state. A Coroner's inquest sat on the body, when, from the evidence, it appears that both men were disposed to relinquish the victory long before it was decided by the death of Fitter, Hill has since declared that he should have 'given in' long before, had his seconds allowed him. Two Hastings, and Hill by Preston and Jackson. The fight was one of the most determined ever witnessed; and at the termination of the 48th round

---

[22] Metastatic cancer: When cancer cells spread from their original location to other parts of the body.

Fitter was taken up lifeless, and his antagonist afterwards carried home in a most dangerous state. A Coroner's inquest sat on the body, when, from the evidence, it appears that both men were disposed to relinquish the victory long before it was decided by the death of Fitter, Hill has since declared that he should have 'given in' long before, had his seconds allowed him. Two surgeons gave it as their opinion that death was occasioned by concussion of the brain, caused by repeated falls. To all outward appearance, however, the survivor was much more punished than his unfortunate antagonist. The jury returned a verdict of manslaughter against Hill, Preston, Jackson, and Hastings. All, with the exception of Hill, who is confined to bed, are yet missing. Preston is known in that part of the country as "The Birmingham Pet," and has fought and won several prize battles. The body-snatchers on Wednesday night, attempted to steal the body of Fitter out of the stable in which it was deposited, but were disappointed, owing to the sudden appearance of the landlord of the public-house, who happened to be up brewing.[23]

Parts of a cadaver, known as "*off cuts*", such as hair and teeth, could be sold for use by wigmakers, and dentists who made the teeth into sets of dentures for wealthy customers:

John Foxley was charged with having on the 20th of July last, violated and disturbed the remains of Jonathan Bedford, who had been buried in St. Bartholomew's Chapel-yard, in the parish of Birmingham. The prisoner, who is an assistant grave-digger, was seen by a little girl, the servant of the sexton, standing by the grave in which the above body had been interred the day before. As no order for the formation of a new grave had been received by the sexton, the conduct of the prisoner excited suspicion; and on the Churchwardens of the parish having been made acquainted with the

---

[23] p.4, *Hereford Journal*, Wednesday 31st March 1830.

circumstance, the grave was examined. The upper part of the lid of the coffin was found open, and the head of the deceased much mutilated; the lower jaw was fractured, and the whole of the teeth in both jaws extracted. Three calendar months in gaol to hard labour. – It is clear from the evidence adduced on the trial, that the object Foxley had in view was not to steal the body, but to extract the teeth, for the purpose of selling them to   the dentists.[24]

St. Bartholomew's was broken into again in 1827:

BODY STEALING.— Edward Calaghan, a decent looking well dressed man from the sister island, only 24 years of age, was indicted for having opened and entered a grave in the burial-ground belonging to St, Bartholemew's chapel in Birmingham, on the 27th of May last, and taken away a dead body intered therein. Mr. GOULBOURN, counsel for the prosecution, said, that the crime of violating the sanctity of the dead, had lately become so frequent in Birmingham, that the authorities of that place had found it necessary to put a stop to it; and there was good reason to believe that bodies were often stolen, mereley for the sake of selling the teeth to the dentists. As there might have been some difficulty in identifying the body to have been that of a particular person the indictment was laid generally and the body was stated to be that of a person unknown. Thomas Taylor said, that at two o'clock in the morning of the 27th of May last, as he was going down Bartholemew-Row, he heard a noise in the chapel yard, and on going up to the wall, he saw the prisoner down upon his knees pushing some shavings into a hamper. The prisoner did not see him, and he knew by the offensive smell what he was about. He looked at the prisoner for a short time, and as he was rising he jumped over the wall and collared him. He asked him if that was his hamper? And he said yes. He then asked the prisoner what he had got there?

---

[24] p.3, *Aris's Birmingham Gazette*, Monday 23rd October 1826.

And he answered he had got some stinking meat, which he had brought out of the market, and he was going to burn it, witness told him that was a very strange place to bring stinking meat. The prisoner then offered to give witness all the money he had to let him go. Witness refused to take his money and called the watchman.— John Little, the watchman, said, Mr. Taylor called him, when he went into the chapel-yard and looked into the hamper; it contained a human body. He said to the prisoner, "It is a pity that a man of your appearance should be found at such work as this." The prisoner replied, "If you were a doctor you would try experiments upon the living." He said, "the law cannot touch me, and I will give you a pound note if you will let me go." The witness told him if he would give him a thousand pounds he would not take it. Thomas Evans the grave digger, said he was called to the chapel yard and searched the hamper, which contained a human body; he went to the burial-ground opposite and found that a grave had been opened, the two ends of the coffin were broken, the lid was split, and the body was taken away. It was the body of a young person, and had been interred nine or ten days. The prisoner, in his defence, said, he was just come into the town, and was going to London on Monday morning. As he was going down the street he saw three men doing something in the chapel-yard and when he went towards them to see what they were about, they all ran away. He then went to search the hamper and as he was going to do, Taylor came and took him. No one saw him go into the ground, or come out of it; he had neither spade nor shovel, and he could not have opened the grave with his hands, for they were as clean then as they were at the present moment. He knew nothing at all of the body; he could not have got it over the wall. Taylor said the prisoner was very dirty particularly his hands, and he smelt very offensively. The burial-ground was on the opposite side of the street, about 15 yards off. The wall was high, with iron railling and one mancould not have got the body over. The jury found him guilty, and the Court sentenced himto be imprisoned six months in the house of correction, and kept to hard labour.[25]

Typically, a member of a grave robbing gang, or his wife, would spend the day loitering in a graveyard waiting for a funeral. The spy would even join the mourners to take careful note of the appearance of the newly dug grave. Alternatively, the gang could be tipped off by informers, usually corrupt sextons, grave diggers (as in the case of John Foxley, above), or undertakers. At night, two members of the gang would appear and, after carefully laying a sheet on the ground, would uncover the head portion of the grave, dumping the loose dirt on the sheet. The body would be pulled from the coffin headfirst with ropes; the shroud was stuffed back into the grave, the lid and the dirt carefully replaced. The process took approximately thirty minutes. The body would then be carried off.

The sexton of Wednesbury church known as "*Ode Picks*" was a notorious resurrectionist supplying the Birmingham anatomists. To catch him in the act the local constabulary left an officer posing as a corpse in his care: while he was removing it from the coffin to his wagon, the "corpse" came to life and arrested him. Brought before the magistrates he pleaded:

Forgive me - I bin a bell-ringer, a psalm-singer at this church for forty 'ear. If yoe'll let me off this time, I'll never rob another stoon, nor touch another boon... (p.84, Hackwood 1924).

Workhouses were also a source of cadavers. Partners of resurrectionists would pose as friends or relatives of dying or dead paupers and claim the corpse, as the following passage testifies from "*The Diary of a Resurrectionist*" by Joshua Naples, a grave digger turned resurrectionist and member of the London Borough

---

[25] p.3, *Birmingham Journal*, Saturday 14th July 1827.

Resurrection Gang[26]:

A favourite trick, in the carrying out of which a woman was generally necessary, was that of claiming the bodies of friendless persons who died in workhouses, or similar institutions. Immediately it was found out that such an one was dead a man and woman, decently clad in mourning, in great grief, and often in tears, called at the workhouse to take away the body of their dear departed relative. If the trick proved successful, as it often did, the body was taken straight off to one of the schools and sold. The parish authorities, probably, were not over particular about giving up the body, if the deceased were a stranger, as by this means they saved the cost of burial. (p.55, Bailey 1896)

Occasionally, corpses would be stolen from family homes where the body had been laid out, prior to burial. One lady, Mrs. Wicks, died on a Monday night and was laid out in her house with two women watching over her. On the Friday night, a man called at the house and convinced the two women to go with him to a nearby public house for a "*comfortable drop*". When they returned to the house it was found the body had been stolen[27].

However, the grave was not always restored: at Tettenhall, near

---

[26] The London Borough Gang, operated from 1802 to 1825. At its peak, it consisted of at least six men, its first leader a former hospital porter named Ben Crouch. Under the protection of Astley Cooper, Crouch's gang supplied some of London's biggest anatomical schools. In 1816, in a dispute over payment, the gang cut off supplies to the St Thomas Hospital Medical School. The school responded by using freelancers, but members of the gang forced their way into the dissecting rooms, threatened the students and attacked the cadavers. The police were called, but concerned about the negative publicity, the school paid the gang's bail and opened negotiations. The gang also put rivals out of business, by desecrating a graveyard - thereby rendering it unsafe to rob graves from for some time- or by reporting freelance resurrectionists to the police (Frank 1976)

[27] p.2, *Staffordshire Advertiser*, Saturday 14th October 1826.

Wolverhampton:

It was discovered, on Friday morning last, that a grave in Tettenhall church-yard had, in the previous night, been disturbed by resurrectionists: the coffin buried therein was wrenched open, and the body it contained appeared to have been taken out, the grave clothes being stripped from it. As the corpse had been buried nine days, it is supposed to have been found in too advanced a state of putrescence to be worth carrying away: it was therefore relaid in its narrow cell, and slightly covered with soil;. No attempt was made to violate any other grave.[28]

It did not prevent the authorities benefiting on occasion:

The body of a pauper buried at Wolverhampton last week, was stolen by the resurrection men, and the overseers of Willenhall, to which parish the pauper had belonged, being determined not to lose the coffin, had it taken from the ground, and offered it for sale. It is now to be seen at a furniture shop in Willenhall and had as a bargain.[29]

If the body was in a less than ideal state it could be abandoned, as in Solihull:

On Sunday, the 7th inst. A great sensation was excited at Solihull by the discovery of a human body, in an advanced state of putrefaction, in a ditch in a field near the residence of Mr. Powell, the discovery was made by a servant lad of that gentleman, and, on the alarm being given, a great concourse of people assembled on the spot, and the body was lifted from the ditch in the presence of the Rev. Archer Clive and several respectable inhabitants of the parish. On being removed to the workhouse, it proved, on

---

[28] p.3, *Staffordshire Advertiser*, Saturday 3rd April 1830.
[29] p.3, *Birmingham Journal*, Saturday 2nd February 1828.

examination, to be the body of a female, but decomposition had taken place to such an extent, as to render it totally impossible to identify the features. The action of the water in which it had laid, had converted the greatest part of the body into adipocere, a substance greatly resembling spermaceti. The body when discovered was enveloped in part of an old coat, and a piece of tattered green baize, and the whole was slightly covered by a few sticks, dry leaves. &c. On Wednesday last, an inquest was held on the body before Mr. Seymour, when, after depositions from Richard Short, Esq. surgeon, and Mr. Powell's servant, the jury returned a verdict of "found dead." Of course, a variety of conjectures have been afloat, but the probability is, that the body was removed from the church yard by resurrectionists, and being found unfit for their purpose was by them left in the place in which it was discovered, where there is every reason to suppose that it has been concealed for several weeks.[30]

In Worcestershire, the body of Hannah Ward, a cook, aged 37 was stolen from Broadway Old Church, in February 1831. The resurrectionists' client refused her body as the legs were decomposing. Rather than being burdened with the body, it was buried in a pile of manure[31].   While a similar occurrence in the village of Grimley resulted in the Churchwardens offering a reward for information regarding the culprits[32]:

ATTEMPT TO ROB A GRAVE!!
In Grimley Church Yard.
FIFTY POUNDS REWARD.
WHEREAS a Shocking Attempt was made on Thursday last night to CARRY AWAY A CORPSE, that had lately been interred in the Church-yard of the Parish of Grimley.

---

[30] p.2, *Birmingham Journal*, Saturday 13th March 1830.
[31] *Worcester News*, Sunday16th January 2022.
[32] p.3, *Worcester Journal*, Thursday 17th October 1822.

This is to give notice that whoever will give information of the person or persons concerned in this horrible affair, shall on his or their conviction receive a Reward of Fifty Pounds from the Churchwardens of Grimley

Trial And Punishment

It was common for the shroud, coffin, and any clothes to be left behind. For example, in 1760, the anatomy professor Robert Robinson (c.1713–1770) of Trinity College, Dublin, on hearing of the death of the Irishman Cornelius Magrath (1736–1760), famed for his height of seven feet three inches, warned his class:

Gentlemen, I have been told that some of you in your zeal have contemplated carrying off the body. I earnestly beg you not to think of such a thing: but if you should be so carried away with your desire for knowledge that thus against my expressed wish you persist in doing so, I would have you remember that if you take only the body, there is no law whereby you can be touched, but if you so much as take a rag or a stocking with it, it is a hanging matter (p.129-30, Kirkpatrick 1912).

The students stole Magrath's corpse from his own wake, leaving behind his clothes and shroud, and swiftly dissected him.

A peculiarity of English law at this time was that to steal a coffin, shroud, or clothing from a corpse was considered a crime against the property of a dead person's heirs and subject to stiff punishment (including hanging), so they were frequently left.

However, a person did not own their own body: it could not be willed as property. Therefore, the theft of a corpse was not considered a felony, only a misdemeanour - unlawful disinterment - for which the punishment was either a fine or imprisonment with hard labour (Hurren 2011; Wise 2004):

RESURRECTION IN COVENTRY.— On Wednesday a considerable sensation was excited throughout Coventry, on it being discovered that some resurrectionists have been availing themselves of the facilities for disinterment which are afforded by the exposed condition of our Church-yard. On opening a grave in the New Church-yard, for the purpose of interring Mr. Robert Cowley, it was discovered that the bodies of two of his children, which had been buried fifteen months ago, had been removed; the linen, caps, and shoes, of the children were left in the coffins, and were in a state of good preservation. Another grave, in which a child belonging to Mrs. Ingram, was interred at the same time, was opened in the evening, when that coffin was also found without the corpse.[33]

In 1827, the Worcestershire Medical and Surgical Society, which included Sir Charles Hastings (1794-1866), the surgeon and founder of the British Medical Association, paid 10 guineas to William Cooke, surgeon of Exeter, who had received a £100 fine for stealing the body and clothes of Elizabeth Taylor from St, David's burial ground *"towards defraying the fine and law expenses incurred by his late prosecution for exhuming a body in furtherance of his anatomical studies."* (p.3, *Worcester Journal*, Thursday 6th September 1827), *"...in testimony of the deep feelings of sorrow with which the society are impressed that so severe a sentence should have been inflicted upon him..."* (p.54, McMenemey 1959).

If a resurrectionist was apprehended it was not necessarily calamitous for him: surgeons protected their resurrectionists. Sir Astley Paston Cooper was so dependent on the *"London Borough Gang"* for cadavers that he exerted his influence to keep them out of jail on numerous occasions, and, if a member was imprisoned, Cooper paid his family a pension while the breadwinner was serving his term (Burch 2007), as did the surgeon Richard Dugard Grainger

---

[33] p.3, *Warwick and Warwickshire Advertiser*, Saturday 11th July 1829.

(1801-1865):

... alone I incurred an expense of 50l. in consequence of allowing [a resurrectionist] *a certain sum per week for two years while he was in prison; during the present season I have expended several guineas in supporting another man's family while he was in prison; these expenses fall, not on the pupils, but on the lecturers ; for if bodies are to be obtained, we must promise to take care of these men when they are in trouble.* (p.45, *Report from the Select Committee on Anatomy* 1828)

This a practice William Sands Cox adhered to, as will be later explored.

If arrested, members of the London Burking Gang had a petition that would be delivered to the heads of the medical and anatomy schools, they supplied:

The humble Petition of John Bishop, and three others,
Most humbly showeth,
That your petitioners have supplied many subjects on various occasions to the several hospitals; and being now in custody, they are conscious in their own minds that they have done nothing more than they have been in the constant habit of doing as resurrectionists, but, being unable to prove their innocence without professional advice, they humbly crave the commiseration of gentlemen who may feel inclined to give some trifling assistance, in order to afford them the opportunity of clearing away the imputation alleged against them. The most trifling sum will be gratefully acknowledged; and your petitioners, as in duty bound, will ever pray. (p.34, Anonymous 1832)

In other words: pay up, or we will cause a scandal.

Transporting The Dead

The stereotypical image of the resurrectionist includes recently disinterred cadavers being placed in a wheelbarrow or handcart and being carried off to the nearest medical school. This was not practical when the nearest school was miles away. It was not unusual for cadavers to be packed up in chests, hampers, or boxes, and sent via mail coaches to the agents of anatomy schools or surgeons. On occasion, details from the coach office or from the destination note could assist in the apprehending of the resurrectionists and/or their customers:

William Simpson, was, on Friday, the 28th ult. Brought before the Magistrates at Lichfield, on a charge of body-snatching. He has been lodging, in company with a female, at the house of Joseph Woolley, in Greenhill, for the last four or five weeks. Another man, of rather respectable appearance, was with them. On Thursday night, about eight o'clock, the two men were seen by Thomas Burton carrying a hamper from the neighbourhood of St. Michael's churchyard to the Swan Inn. His suspicions were excited, and, upon application to the proper authorities, the hamper was ordered to be opened, and found to contain the body of Joseph Slater, which had been interred on the Tuesday previous. The hamper was directed, "Mr. Johnson, care of Messrs. Neel and Hill, No. 178, Tooley-street, Southwark, London." At the prisoner's lodgings two pairs of trowsers, dirtied with clay, were found. His companion paid the booking of the hamper, which was left at the door of the coach office by the prisoner. He was apprehended by Mr. John Burton. The prisoner was committed,— It is feared that the prisoner and his companion have been carrying on their depredations in this neighbourhood extensively, as we hear the body of a child, of Mr. Claridge, of Stowe-street, which was buried on Wednesday week, has been stolen. Suspicion was first excited by the sexton of St. Michael's having, on Tuesday, observed that three graves, which he had a day or two before banked up afresh, had been disturbed. On examination, it was found that the coffins in two of them had been broken open; but the bodies being in an advanced state of decomposition, were not, it seems, thought fit subjects for surgical operations, and therefore left behind. In the third grave the coffin remained secure. It is supposed, that when the resurrectionists saw the date of the decease of the person it contained, they desisted from their undertaking. The most recently buried corpse of the three had been interred about six weeks and the fellows were deceived by the fresh appearance of the graves.[34]

Simpson and his accomplice, James King, were each fined £10 and sentenced to ten months imprisonment[35]. *"Neel and Hill"* were William Neale and Richard Hale, Chemists and Druggists, of 178 Tooley Street (*London Morning Herald*, Monday 28th June 1830, p.8). *"Johnson"* may have been an employee of the nearby hospitals of St. Thomas or Guys.

Resurrectionists at Stafford.— A few days ago, a large square box was brought, by a country man, in a wheelbarrow, to the George Inn, in this town, to be forwarded by the first coach to London. Some suspicion was excited respecting its contents; but Mr. R. Jones thought it better to write to a police-officer in London, to take such steps there as might be requisite, rather than to open the box here. He accordingly wrote to Bow-street; and one of the officers attended at the inn where the coach stopped, and found the box, which he immediately opened, and discovered in it a human body! A man called for the box, who offered to take the officer to the person who had employed him to fetch it away. Whilst the officer was absent, on a wrong scent, the box was called for, and no further tidings have been heard of it or the parties.[36]

---

[34] p.4, *Staffordshire Advertiser*, Saturday 6th December 1828.
[35] p.4, *Staffordshire Advertiser*, Saturday 17th January 1829.
[36] p.4, *Staffordshire Advertiser*, Saturday 30th October 1830.

RESURRECTIONISTS.— Two resurrectionists have been apprehended at Hereford.—On Saturday morning a hamper was delivered at the Champion coach-office, Hereford, to Mr. J. Bosley, jun. a son of one of the coach-proprietors, to be sent to London. Mr.B. suspecting that it contained stolen goods, sent for Mr. Howells, one of the city police, who opened it, and discovered that it contained a body, which was afterwards proved to be that of an old pensioner named Hardman, who was buried in the burial ground of All Saints on the 31st ult. It was soon discovered that two men had been engaged intaking up the body, and they were both taken into custody. The sensation caused in the city and neighbourhood by the discovery of this transaction, has been much increased by a remark of Mr. John Bosley, jun., who, on the inquest, stated that during the winter many similar packages had passed through the Champion coach-office. It has since been discovered that the body of Mrs. Lee, wife of Mr. Lee, tailor, had been stolen from St. John's church-yard. Since this discovery Mr. Lee has been dangerously ill. Besides the above two men, two persons named Phillips and Closs have been taken up, on suspicion of being connected with the resurrectionists; Closs stated himself to be the servant of a Mr. Parks, who has lately taken a house near Hereford, but formerly (it is said) resided at Worcester. The Hereford Journal states that Parks is not to be found; he had obtained goods of many persons, some of whom have succeeded in getting them back again.[37]

Due to high demand, the trade in cadavers had reached massive proportions. The numbers being transported around the country meant ships had to be utilized, which could result in macabre consequences. Such as the incident in Liverpool, reported

---

[37] p.3, *Worcester Journal*, Thursday 12th January 1832.

in the *Staffordshire Advertiser*:[38]

WHOLESALE RESURRECTIONISTS

Instances of the disinterment of one or two human bodies, for the purposes of dissection, have occasionally come within our knowledge, in this town, as well as in others; but it would seem, by a discovery made on Tuesday, that there has existed an organized company of resurrectionists in Liverpool, for the purpose of the medical students of Edinburgh with subjects for dissection upon a large scale. The following is an account of the circumstances connected with this extraordinary affair, which is altogether unparalleled in this town, and has, of course, produced a strong excitement of feeling, and an unpleasant sensation amongst all classes of the community. It appears that, on Monday afternoon, three casks were sent to be shipped on board the Latona Smack, Captain Walker, who was taking in goods for Leith, in George's Dock Passage. They had been Newfoundland oil casks, and were marked on the outside "Bitter Salts," and accompanied by a shipping note, of which the following is a copy:

"Please ship on board the Latona three casks of Bitter Salts, from Mr. Brown, Agent, Liverpool, to Mr. G. H. Ironson, Edinburgh.

"J.Brown."

"Liverpool, Oct.9, 1826."

"To the Carron Company"

The casks were put down betwixt decks, to be stowed away in their proper place the following morning. Before this was accomplished, the men employed in moving them were much annoyed by an offensive smell which proceeded from the casks, and informed the captain of this circumstance. Upon a closer examination, the Captain found a small hole in one of the casks, stopped up with a whisp of hay, and, upon drawing it out, the stench

---

[38] p.4, *Staffordshire Advertiser*, Saturday 14th October 1826.

became almost intolerable. He then started one of the bungs, and upon putting his hand into the hole, found, to his utter surprise, that the contents of the casks were human bodies. Assured of this fact, he hastened to communicate the same to his owners, the Carron Company, in Redcross-street. The respectable agent of that establishment promptly apprised the police of the discovery, who had the casks immediately conveyed to the dead-house [mortuary], *in Chapel-street, where the*

contents were examined, and found to consist of eleven human bodies, entirely bestrewed with and packed in salt.

The carter who had been employed to bring down the casks for shipment in the Latona, having stated where he brought them from, a party of the police were sent to examine and bring away the remaining contents of the cellar in Hope-street. Upon their arrival they found several casks and sacks full of dead bodies, which were brought down to the dead-house, and underwent an examination by Mr. Davis, surgeon, and the contents (including those in the casks taken from on board the vessel) found to amount to the extraordinary number of thirty-three human bodies, of both sexes, and of various ages. It is almost superfluous to observe, that the business of examining the half-putrid bodies (which were, doubtless, intended for dissection in Edinburgh) was attended with a stench, almost impossible to be borne by the parties who were obliged to assist in the revolting service. The person under whose premises this wholesale charnel-house had, unfortunately, been formed, is a gentleman of respectability and character, and will doubtless, be able to clear himself from any imputation of connivance to the business. It would appear that the disgraceful traffic has been carried on for a considerable time, but by whom, remains yet to be ascertained; and we much fear, that the publicity which has already been given to this affair, will greatly contribute to defeat the efforts which are now making to bring the delinquents to justice.

The following particulars transpired in the court of examination in the Police Office, held before Richard Bellin, Esq.

Coroner:

*Robert Boughey, a police-officer, deposed that this morning, (Tuesday) in consequence of a notice sent from the carron Company's office, he went to the smack Latona, lying in George's Dock passage, and there found three casks, which had been brought to the vessel on Monday afternoon, and which, on examination, he found to contain dead human bodies; he immediately had them conveyed to the dead-house in Chapel-street. Deponent succeeded in finding the carter, George Leech, who had brought them down. Leech told him that he got them from a cellar in Hope-street, where there were several other casks of a similar description. Deponent, accompanied by several other officers and the carter, immediately proceeded to Hope-street, when Leech pointed out a cellar under the Rev. James M*Gowan's school-room, as the place from whence he got his load. Deponent accordingly went to Mr. McGowan, and inquired for the key, for the purpose of examining the cellar, but was informed by that gentleman that he had not got it, having let the cellar, in January last, to a man who said his name was John Henderson, a cooper, and a native of Greenock. Under these circumstances deponent broke open the door, when he found a number of casks, three of which were filled with dead bodies, all ready for embarkation, and the remainder (with the exception of two which were filled with salt) empty; besides which, he found three sacks, each containing dead bodies, and several canvass dresses, the exception of two which were filled with salt) empty; besides which, he found three sacks, each containing dead bodies, and several canvass dresses, very dirty, which were hanging up, supposed to have been worn by the miscreants in their nightly employment. He caused the whole of the articles to be put into a cart and conveyed to the dead-house.*

George Leech, a carter, deposed, that on Monday afternoon, between three and four o'clock, he was with his brother's cart at the Dry Dock, when a tall stout man, with black whiskers and with a Scotch accent, asked him what he would charge to cart three casks from Hope-street, to the George Dock Passage; deponent agreed for sixpence in addition, "to be careful in putting the casks down on the quay." He (deponent) took them, as he was directed, to the Latona, lying in the George's Dock Passage, and delivered the note to the mate, who returned it saying he must take it to the office in Redcross-street. He took the note and left it on the counter. He then put the casks on the quay which were afterwards put between decks.

The casks were directed "Mr. G. H. Ironson, Edinburgh." He is sure that the casks which were seized by Boughey, are the same which he carted down.

Thomas William Davis, surgeon, deposed, that he went to the dead-house, in Chapel-street, where he found the three casks which had been seized by Boughey; he immediately opened them and found them to contain dead human bodies in salt. The first cask contained one man and two women; the second, two men and two women; the third, three men and one woman. The cart containing the casks and sacks brought from the cellar soon after arrived. In three casks and three sacks he found nine men, five women, five boys, and three girls. Total number of bodies 33. The bodies were all whole and in a perfect state. Those in the casks appeared to have been dead six or seven days; those in the sacks might have been dead two or three days. The whole of the bodies were entirely naked; there was not the least mark of any eternal violence on them; nor was there any reason to suppose that the persons had not died a natural death. Deponent supposed, from the circumstance of discovering the remains of a thread on the toes of one of the young women, (which practice is used, in some families, to keep the feet of the deceased persons together), that the bodies had been disinterred.

At the suggestion of Mr. Davis, who stated that several of the bodies were far gone in a state of decomposition, the Coroner immediately issued his warrant for their interment, which was accordingly carried into execution on Tuesday.

From the various materials found in the cellar, it may be conjectured that the bodies had, in the first process, been put into a strong brine, and afterwards, when thoroughly pickled, packed in the casks with the dry salt. Amongst other articles was a large brass syringe, which might, probably, have been employed in ejecting a preservative liquid into the veins of the "subjects".

The question must be asked: how many bodies were ferried along the canals of the West Midlands, not just to the anatomy schools and teaching hospitals of the Midlands, but also to those of London?

More than once, large shipments of bodies from the public graveyards in Ireland and other countries, packed in piano cases and kegs were left unclaimed on the docks of Liverpool and London: which did not fail to attract the attention of the authorities (Guttmacher 1935). For example, the *Wolverhampton Chronicle and Staffordshire Advertiser* reported that: "*A vessel recently sailed from Ostend, with a cargo of dead bodies, intended for the London resurrectionists*".[39]

The Resurrectionists

The most infamous – and well-known - resurrectionists are those who have murdered.

In 1828, William Burke and William Hare murdered sixteen people in Edinburgh and sold the bodies to the surgeon Dr. Robert Knox. Their method of murdering, using suffocation, became known as "*Burking*". When caught, in return for immunity, Hare turned King's evidence against Burke, who was sentenced to be executed. Following his execution in 1829, Burke was publicly dissected in the anatomy theatre of Edinburgh University's Old College, and parts of his skin were used to make wallets, calling card cases and to bind books. His skeleton is on display at the University of Edinburgh's Anatomy Museum. The fate of Hare is unknown.

---

[39] p.3 *Wolverhampton Chronicle and Staffordshire Advertiser*, Wednesday, 20th January 1830

(Dudley-Edwards 2014). Dr. Knox was cleared of complicity by a committee of inquiry who reported that they had "*seen no evidence that Dr Knox or his assistants knew that murder was committed in procuring any of the subjects brought to his rooms*" (p.572, *London Medical Gazette*). There was a public outcry: in February 1829, a crowd gathered outside his house and burned an effigy of him, and numerous caricatures lampooned him. He was shunned by the medical establishment but continued to teach and write. He died in London in 1862 (Rosner 2010).

In London in 1831, the three resurrectionists: John Bishop, Thomas Williams, and James May, drugged and murdered three people including a 14-year-old Italian boy named Carlo Ferrari. The victims' bodies were sold to anatomists and surgeons from St Bartholomew's Hospital, St Thomas's Hospital, and King's College in London. Bishop and Williams were executed, and their bodies dissected by surgeons. They became known as the "*Italian Boy murderers*" or the "*London Burkers*" (Wise 2004).

Also, in London in 1831, Catherine Walsh of Whitechapel who made her living by selling laces and cotton, was murdered by Elizabeth Ross, who sold the body to surgeons. Ross was hanged for murder (Anonymous 1832; Donneley 2007).

Several resurrectionists operated around the West Midlands.

Hackwood (1924) reports that in 1826, Daniel Stone was convicted of disturbing a grave at Upper Gornal. As punishment he was tied to a cart and dragged along the road from Sedgley to Bilston, being whipped as he went. In 1828, Thomas Stokes was arrested on the suspicion of having been engaged in grave robbing in the churchyards around Wolverhampton. Described as a "*rogue and a vagabond*" by the magistrate Rev. William Leigh of Bilston, he was sentenced to two months hard labour at the treadmill[40,41].

---

[40] The treadmill had steps set into two cast iron wheels. These drove a shaft that could be used to mill corn, pump water, or connect to a large fan for resistance.
[41] p.3, *Worcester Journal*, Thursday 27th October 1831.

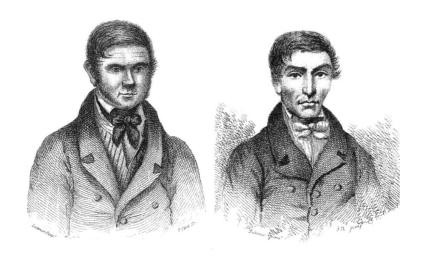

William Burke   William Hare
Both by George Andrew Lutenor (1829)

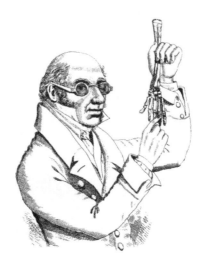

Dr. Robert Knox
Unknown Artist

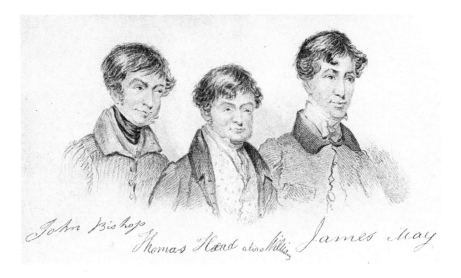

John Bishop, Thomas Williams, and James May
The Italian Boy Murderers/ The London Burkers
(Wellcome Images)

There is some irony in this. During the Cholera[42]pandemic of 1832, the Rev. Leigh headed the relief effort in Bilston and had to enlist the help of Sands Cox, the main patron of the resurrectionists in the area (Goodman 2023).

On occasion, being related to a resurrectionist could land a person in trouble:

A young man of this city [Worcester] *was apprehended near the burial-ground belonging to the House of Industry* [Workhouse], *at a very early hour on Sunday morning, under the suspicion of being a "body snatcher." He was examined before the Magistrates on Monday, when he confessed, that, being intoxicated, he was induced by two men from London (one of whom was his brother to go to the burial-ground, with the view of stealing bodies; they took with them two spades, bags, &c. but just as they were going to commence operations) some persons coming by, suspecting what their object was, seized the prisoner, but the others made off, leaving the spades, &c. behind them. They have not since been heard of. The prisoner, who previously bore a good character was discharged.*[43]

The most prolific resurrectionists in the West Midlands were Joseph Grainger and John Watts.

Joseph Grainger of Birmingham

Aside from his career as a resurrectionist, Grainger, or Chapman, (a name he sometimes used), had served two months imprisonment with hard labour for keeping a disorderly house, (i.e. brothel), in Chapel Street, Birmingham in July 1827[44]. In November 1827, Grainger was apprehended by armed guards attempting to

---

[42] Cholera: caused by an infection of the bacterium Vibrio cholerae. Symptoms include large amounts of watery diarrhoea lasting a few days, vomiting and muscle cramps and can prove fatal.

[43] p.3, *Worcester Journal*, Thursday 27th October 1831.

[44] p.3 *Birmingham Journal*, Saturday 14th July 1827.

steal a cadaver from Aston churchyard, Birmingham[45]:

Since it has been known that a gang of these respectable characters have been in the neighbourhood, a degree of vigilance has been aroused among the grave diggers, sextons, &c, of the church yards around Birmingham; and various rumours have been afloat of the successful attacks made by the body snatchers. On Saturday last suspicion having been excited by the appearance of some strangers about the church yard of Aston, during the time of the interment of an aged and respectable inhabitant of Deritend, [Mrs. Russell] a watch of three men was appointed for the ensuing night, armed with bludgeons, swords, &c. The hour of three on the following morning had arrived without any appearance of the professional gentlemen from the metropolis, but shortly after, slowly and silently were perceived creeping along towards the new made grave, four men armed, with their implements of trade, who immediately began to work. Upon stopping for a short time, one of them said, "It's all right." When the three men in ambush rushed from behind an adjoining tombstone, and a scuffle commenced, which ended in one of the men being apprehended, and very much bruised. He was immediately conveyed to the prison in Bordesley; and on Monday brough before the magistrates at our public office; but as the investigation took place in the private room, we are unable to state more at the proceedings than that the man was discharged...

Further details concerning Grainger's discharge were soon forthcoming due to local outrage[46]:

In consequence of information received from the prison-keeper of Bordesley, that a man had been given into custody on charge of

---

[45] p.3, *Birmingham Journal*, Saturday 8th December 1827.
[46] p.3, *Birmingham Journal*, Saturday 15th December 1827.

*attempting to dig up the body of a respectable inhabitant of
Deritend, from Aston church-yard, some of the friends of the
deceased attended the Public-Office on the following Monday, Dec.
3rd, for the purpose of hearing the examination. They were surprised
at being informed by the prison-keeper, that he had received an
order to discharge the man, no public examination having taken
place. On referring to one of the magistrates, it was answered, that
the man was charged with no offence, and that a hearing could
not be granted. After some debate between the churchwardens of
Aston and the relatives of the deceased, one of the clerks of the office
was consulted on the subject, by the parties concerned, and the facts
being stated to him, he said, that the attempt to commit a
misdemeanour was a misdemeanour itself; that the accused being
caught in the church-yard at an unseasonable hour, and with tools
in his hands working at the head of a newly made grave, was
sufficient evidence of his intentions. A message was then sent to the
magistrates, by the friends of the deceased and the churchwardens
of Aston, purporting that it was their opinion that the magistrates
had not done their duty in discharging the prisoner without an
examination, and that the evidence ought to be heard. This was at
length acceded to, and an examination took place in the private
room. The evidence given against the prisoner was to the following
purport. Having suspicions of an intended attempt of the
resurrectionists (since two bodies were stolen from that place a
short time before) two men kept a watch in the belfry of Aston
church-yard, on Friday night, Nov. 30. About a quarter past one on
Saturday morning, a man was observed to steal quietly through the
church-yard towards a grave, where a person had been buried the
morning before; and shortly afterwards two more came, having a
squat box, a spade, ropes, sack. &c.− One of them knelt down and
began to throw out the earth from the grave as quickly as he could.
Upon this the men who were watching them, approached from
different sides, and while the attention of the resurrectionists was
taken up by the one, the other came upon them from behind,*

unawares, struck the prisoner who was digging, on the head with a sword, and after a short scuffle took him together with the box, sack, ropes, spade, &c. which they had brought and set beside the grave. The other two men escaped. About a wheelbarrow full of earth had been thrown out. The prisoner was asked his name, he said it was Chapman, but he was more known by the name of Grainger. One of the magistrates said that the watch had done very right in apprehending the prisoner, but, at the same time, there was no evidence on which he could be committed, as the body had not been removed, He was accordingly discharged.

The man who had apprehended Grainger was Robert Roberts, the Parish Clerk[47]. The Churchwardens of Aston were determined to ensure Grainger was prosecuted and the following appeal was issued in March 1828[48]:

A BODY-STEALER.
FIVE POUNDS REWARD.
WHEREAS, at the last Quarter Sessions, held for the county of Warwick, a true bill was found against JOSEPH CHAPMAN, better known by the name of Grainger, for a misdemeanour in attempting to steal a DEAD BODY out of the Church-yard of the Parish of Aston, near Birmingham – Churchwardens of the said parish hereby offer a reward of THREE POUNDS upon his apprehension, and a further sum of TWO POUNDS to be paid upon his conviction.

The said JOSEPH CHAPMAN is about 44 years of age, stands five feet five inches high, with a pale complexion, long visage, brown hair, and slender make; has a thin nose marked with the small-pox. Some time back he lived in Lawrence-street, but after he was taken in the act of committing the above offence he removed to Nineveh, and is supposed to be in that neighbourhood..

Vestry-room, Aston Church, March 5, 1828.

---

[47] p.2, *Aris's Birmingham Gazette*, Monday 21st July 1828.
[48] p.3, *Aris's Birmingham Gazette*, Monday 21st July 1828.

In October 1828, Grainger and his accomplice John Watts (using the alias Pointon), were caught stealing the body of Richard Clark, from Tipton churchyard and were tried at Staffordshire Assizes[49].

RESURRECTIONISTS.

John Watts, aged 21, and Joseph Grainger, aged 45, were tried on an indictment charging them with having disinterred and exposed the body of Richard Clark, which had been buried in the churchyard of Tipton, in this county.

From the evidence of Isaac Clark, the father of the "subject" of this prosecution, it appeared that his son died on the 16th of October. Last, and was buried on the 19th.

On the night of the 20th about 10 o'clock, James Murphy, an Irishman, who resides in Sedgley, was passing Tipton churchyard. It being a clear moonlight night, he saw two men, one standing on the wall, the other standing on a bench behind the wall, and a naked human body lying on the wall. Being alarmed at seeing two men engaged in such a transaction, he durst not approach them, but he kept at the distance of 10 yards, but in order to apprise them that someone was near, he coughed, and then the man upon the wall let the body fall inside the wall. Murphy made the best of his way to the Curate's house to inform him, "thinking" as he said, "that those who would steal the dead, would kill the living."

When he returned with the minister, and a person named Redding, the men were gone, having taken the body with them. They then went into the church to watch, and taking out a pane of glass they saw the prisoners enter a field adjoining the churchyard, and drag the body from under a bush down the field. They then left the church and pursued them, but did not overtake them.

A miner, named Brown, seeing Watts running from the churchyard about one o'clock in the morning, seized him, and

---

[49] p.3, *Staffordshire Advertiser*, Saturday 24th January 1829.

afterwards delivered him up to the constable.

Grainger was taken about 4 o'clock the same morning, by an engineer, named Job Dudley, who saw him come from a bush about 60 yards from the Horseley Colliery; before he apprehended him, he enquired where he had been all night; at first he said at the engine, pointing to one near; afterwards he said he came from Birmingham. Dudley then suspected him, (having heard of the transaction,) and told him he thought he was one, and took him into custody. There were two shovels and a grafting tool found near the place where Grainger was taken.

The identity of the body was proved by the father, who very feelingly said, "when I saw it I knew it was my son."

The identity of the prisoners as provided by Murphy, and several other witnesses.

The fact was indirectly proved by the prisoner watts, who on his way to prison claimed a cart which was found in a field near the churchyard, which contained a box, a waist-coat, and some straw; there was also a horse in the field, ready harnessed, but no one claimed that.

After all the witnesses had been examined, Watts requested that they might be re-called, which was done, and they were severally cross-examined by him, but nothing could be proved in favour of the prisoners.

No persons appeared to their characters.

Mr. WILLIAMS, (Counsel for Grainger,) who had cross-examined each of the witnesses with great discrimination, addressed the Jury on his behalf, and besought them to dismiss from their minds that prejudice which at all times existed in cases of this kind, but which had become stronger and more universal than ever under the excitement of recent revolting transactions [Burke and Hare murders]. *He reminded them of the evident eagerness with which the witnesses had given their evidence, and their great apparent anxiety to convict. The Irishman (Murphy,) who had adopted the truly Hibernian expedient of coughing that he might not be seen,*

(Laughter) had decidedly shewn this feeling, and he really thought his evidence should be very cautiously received. As to the identity of Grainger, he thought there were doubts, of which he ought to have the benefit, and receive from them a verdict of acquittal.

The Jury found both the prisoners guilty.

SIR OSWALD MOSLEY[50] previous to passing sentence observed, that the offence of which they were found guilty, was too common in this country, and one which it was the duty of the magistrates to suppress, and he regretted that the law did not empower them to pass a heavier sentence than six months imprisonment, and a fine of £10 each to the King.

It was originally – incorrectly – believed that Grainger had escaped prosecution for grave robbing in Aston due to "*an excellent character* [reference] *from some of the surgeons of this town*"[51]. However, following his and Watts' arrest in Tipton, documents in the National Archives reveal that a petition pleading leniency was sent to Robert Peel[52], the Home Secretary, signed by several medical men including William Sands Cox of the Birmingham School of Medicine. The prison records describe the two prisoners as "*Medical*

---

[50] Sir Oswald Mosley (1785-1871): 2nd Baronet of Ancoats. Member of Parliament for Portarlington (1806-7), Winchelsea (1807-12), Midhurst (1817-18), and North Staffordshire (1832-37) and High Sheriff for Staffordshire (1814). He wrote several local and natural history books, including *'History of the Castle, Priory and Town of Tutbury'* (1832) and *'Natural History of Tutbury'* (1863).

[51] p.3, *Birmingham Journal*, Saturday 8th December 1827

[52] Sir Robert Peel (1788 –1850), was a British Conservative statesman who served twice as Prime Minister (1834–1835, 1841–1846), while simultaneously serving as Chancellor of the Exchequer (1834–1835), and twice as Home Secretary (1822–1827, 1828–1830). He is regarded as the father of modern British policing, owing to his founding of the Metropolitan Police Service.

Students":

> *School of Medicine and Surgery,*
> *Birmingham, March 6ᵗʰ 1829*

Sir –

We the undersigned lecturers of the School of Medicine respectfully beg leave to submit to your consideration the following case-

John Watts and Joseph Grainger charged with having disinterred the body of Richard Clarke from the burial ground of Tipton were sentenced at the Stafford Quarter sessions held on the 16 of January to six months imprisonment and to pay a fine of 10£ each – John Watts has already been confined in gaol from October, both men are married, Grainger has a young family. Under these circumstances as the legislature as yet affords no protection, no means to cultivate the science of anatomy; and the regulations of the Royal College of Surgeons compel the medical student to prosecute dissections we humbly trust you will be pleased to mitigate the sentence.

We have the honour to continue your most obedient humble servants.

Richard Pearson M.D.
John K. Booth M.D.
John Eccles M.D.
Alfred Jukes, Surgeon
William Sands Cox Surgeon
To the Right Honourable Robert Peel
Secretary of State[53]

There is no record of the sentence or fine being waived. The medical school probably paid the fine and ensured the prisoners' families were financially secure. It should also be noted that Robert

---

[53] National Archives: Prisoner name: John Watts and Joseph Grainger. Prisoner occupation: Medical students. HO 17/113/18

Peel was one of the Patrons of the Birmingham School of Medicine and Surgery (see page 17).

On January 29th, 1830, Mary Oliver of Henley-in-Arden, Warwickshire, "*a fine grown married woman, about 30 years of age*"[54] was found dead in her bed. It was decided she had "*died by the visitation of God*"[55] and interred in the Parish churchyard at Wootten Wawen. However, the clerk, having seen "*some suspicious looking persons about on the day of the funeral*"[56], guards were posted for four nights. Unfortunately, her body was stolen three weeks later. It soon reappeared:

THE RESURRECTIONISTS DISAPPOINTED.—*Considerable excitement has prevailed at Northfield, a village in this neighbourhood, during the past week, owing to a dead body being left at one of the Inns, packed up in a wooden box, directed for London. On Monday last, a man named Chambers, a potatoe dealer of this town, called at the Bell at Northfield with his cart, and left the case, with instructions that it should be forwarded to the place of its destination, either by coach or caravan. The people of the house, however, kept the package until Wednesday, when suspicion was awoke by noisome smells proceeding from its interior. Information of the circumstance was conveyed to the Rev. J.T. Fenwick, a resident magistrate, and the box, we believe, upon his authority, was immediately opened. It was found to contain the body of a woman, who upon enquiry. Proved to be the wife of the hostler at the White Swan in Henley, and who had been interred at the church of the latter village, the Monday week before. A few days after the funeral of the deceased, several very suspicious characters were seen in the neighbourhood, which led to her husband watching*

---

[54] p.3, *Warwick and Warwickshire Advertiser*, Saturday 13th March 1830.
[55] *Warwick and Warwickshire Advertiser op cit*
[56] *Warwick and Warwickshire Advertiser* op *cit*

very closely the ground in which she was interred. The night, however, before the corpse was stolen from the grave, Chambers called at the White Swan with his horse and cart, and after baiting, presented the husband with the usual fee given to hostlers on such occasions. Little did he know, or suspect, the object of the donor's visit. The following morning it was discovered that the grave had been opened, and the body stolen; though the thieves had taken the greatest pains to remove all outward trace of violence to the ground, and beneath the sod had placed straw to impede the entrance of the spade. It appears that the body was subsequently brought to Birmingham; but what could be the object of Chambers in conveying the booty to Northfield, it is impossible to conjecture. The directions of the passage was," To George Pilcher, Esq. 28 Dean-street, Southwark, London." Immediately the contents of the box were known, steps were taken to apprehend Chambers, but he has hitherto eluded the vigilance of the police. An inquest sat upon the body, at Northfield, yesterday, but with its decision we are as yet unacquainted. We learn, however, that the deceased died very suddenly, and before her interment a coroner's investigation took place, the result of which was, a verdict to the effect that she "died by the visitation of God." The men seen in Henley and the neighbourhood, at the time of the funeral, and who aroused the suspicions of the husband, have not been since seen[57].

The address to where the body was to be sent, *"Pilcher, 35, Dean-street, London"* belonged to George Pilcher (1801–1855). an English aural surgeon, later fellow of the Royal College of Surgeons of England and lecturer on surgery (*Dictionary of National Biography*).

A local man, John Wickham, was apprehended in connection with the robbery and taken to Warwick gaol where he confessed to

---

[57] p.2, *Birmingham Journal*, Saturday 27th February 1830.

having two accomplices: Chambers, and Grainger[58,59]. Grainger was arrested on the 18th of March while out walking with his wife in Sun Street, Edgbaston, by Officer Hall and taken to Henley to be questioned by the magistrates[60]. Wickham appeared at Warwick Crown Court[61]:

CROWN COURT

STEALING A BODY.—John Wickhan, a foolish stupid looking fellow about 21 years of age, was indicted for stealing the body of Mary Oliver, out of a grave in the church-yard of Wootton Wawen, on the 18th of February last. There was nothing scarcely to connect the prisoner with this offence, excepting his own confession before the committing Magistrates.

Joseph Oliver, the husband of the deceased, said that his wife died on the 29th of January, and was buried in Wootten Wawen church yard, on the 1st of February. He paid some men to watch the grave for four nights, and on the fifth night the body was removed. He saw the body afterwards at the Bell at Northfield, where it had been left in a box directed to somebody in London. On the Sunday night before the body was stolen, the prisoner was at the White Swan at Henley. On the night the body was stolen, an old man called at the Swan with a grey horse and cart, and about nine left and went toward Wootton.

The box containing the body was left at the Bell, by a man by the name of Chambers, who brought it there in a cart, drawn by a grey horse. The box, on the day after it was left, was opened by a constable.

The prisoner confessed, when he was committed, that he met

---

58 p.3, *Worcester Journal*, Thursday 25th March 1830.
59 p.4, *Worcester Herald*, Saturday 10th April 1830.
60 p.3, *Birmingham Journal*, Saturday 17th April 1830.
61 p.4, *Worcester Herald*, Saturday 10th April 1830.

two men at Birmingham, one of the name of Grainger, and the other of the name of Chambers, who asked them to go with them to Hanley. They there sent him to buy a shovel, and then took him to Wootton church-yard. When they had taken up the body, at a given signal he took a bag, helped them to drag the body out of the grave, and put it into the cart.

When they got into the road, they gave him 14s. [shillings] *and he went away.*

The Jury found him Guilty and sentenced him to six calendar months hard labour.

There is no record of Grainger or Chambers being charged.

Grainger was arrested again, in October 1831, together with Benjamin Sandbrook, after stealing the body of John Fenton from the   chapel yard at Smethwick[62]:

CONVICTION OF RESURRECTIONISTS

Benjamin Sandbrook (aged 30,) and Joseph Grainger (50,) were indicted for breaking and entering the chapel yard of Smethwick, in the parish of Harborne, on the 31st of Oct. 1831, and disinterring and taking away the body of John Fenton, which had been interred there.

Mr. WHATELEY conducted the case for the prosecution. He briefly stated the facts he was about to prove in evidence; and observed that Sandbrook was taken into custody with the body in his possession, and therefore the Jury could not entertain a doubt of his guilt; against Grainger the evidence would not be so strong, and yet, he thought, it would be sufficiently so to warrant a verdict of guilty. He then called:

Abraham Darby, a labourer, who deposed that he remembered being near the Birmingham canal, near Saturday Bridge, at half-

---

[62] p.3, *Staffordshire Advertiser*, Saturday 14th January 1832.

past five o'clock on the morning of the 31st of October last. Saturday Bridge is on the way from Smethwick towards Birmingham. Smethwick is in the parish of Harborne, and three miles from Birmingham. At the time mentioned, he saw the prisoner Sandbrook, with a wheelbarrow, containing a bag, covered with green baize. Witness said "Mind, where are you going with that barrow?"

Sandbrook made him no answer. Witness had some suspicion, followed him, and repeated his question, and also asked him where his home was? He replied in "Womble" lane. Witness said that was no road to Womble Lane. Witness than asked him what he had got in that barrow? Sandbrook replied "Nothing at all, belonging to nobody but himself." Witness then said he insisted upon knowing, and called to Joseph Underhill, to take Sandbrook into Welch's lock-house yard. The barrow was then searched, and in the bag was found a corpse – the body of a man. Witness took the prisoner and the body to Birmingham. The next day, witness observed dirt and soil upon Sandbrook, halfway up the leg. At the time he first saw Sandbrook, he saw another man about 10 or 18 yards before him.

Cross-examined by MR. CORBETT, (Counsel for Grainger.) The other man was walking along the road by the canal side. He did not run away.

Joseph Underhill corroborated the latter part of Darby's evidence.

Job Fenton (the son of the deceased person, whose body was found in the bag) proved that he had the misfortune to lose his father in October last. On the 30th of October, he was buried in Smethwick church-yard. Witnesses attended his funeral. The body found in the bag was shewn to him next morning. It was his father's body. Sandbrook came to see his father before his death, and during his illness.

Thomas Scott, constable of Smethwick, said that on the 1st of November he apprehended Grainger in his own home in Birmingham. He took Sandbrook and Grainger into the parlour together; and asked Grainger if he knew Sandbrook? He replied he *had never seen him in his life before. Sandbrook said "Did not I dine with you on Sunday upon pork?" Grainger declared that he had not. Sandbrook said "Be'n't those the half-boots you lent me, to go and fetch the corpse in?" Grainger said "No: he never saw him of the boots in his life."*

Nothing important was elicited on Scott's cross-examination.

Charles Heamhurst, constable of Smethwick, proved that on Wednesday the 2nd of November, he searched Grainger's house, and there he found a coat, which he now produced. [The coat was very much soiled, particularly the sleeves.] The soil then appeared fresh. Witness knows the sort of soil in Smethwick church-yard: it is a gravelly soil, like that with which the coat was soiled.

Thomas Jones, a metal roller, of Birmingham, proved that he was a lodger at Grainger's house some weeks before the 31st of October. His house was on the canal side between Snow-hill and Wombourne. He remembered Grainger being apprehended on this charge. On the Sunday before that day, he remembered Sandbrook coming to the house. He had often seen him there before. Sandbrook dined that day at Grainger's house. He sat at a table by himself. After dinner, witness went out, and returned again about the hour of ten at night. He found Grainger and Sandbrook in the house when he returned. They were sitting together. Shortly afterwards, they both went out of the house: one went first, and the other followed. They were out about a minute, and then returned. When they came back again, Grainger desired witness to go to bed. Witness did not immediately go, and Grainger again told him to go to bed. Witness went to bed between 10 and 11, and soon after heard the outer door open and shut again. He did not hear anything of Sandbrook and Grainger after that time. [Here the coat, produced by Heamhurst to be Grainger's coat. He was in the habit of wearing a coat of that colour and kind. He could not swear positively that it was Grainger's coat. No other man lived in the house at that time, except himself and Grainger. It was not his (witness's coat). There were wheel-barrows about Grainger's premises; but he did not observe one there that week.

Cross-examined. Witness could not swear that it was Grainger's coat. Grainger kept a public house. All that he knew about Sandbrook being there was that he was there sometimes as other customers were, and that he dined there on the Sunday by himself.

Re-examined.—Before the magistrates, witness had said that the coat was Grainger's coat. He had no doubt now that it was Grainger's coat.

William Welsh, the keeper of a beer-shop, in Hospital-street, Birmingham, proved that Sandbrook and Grainger were at his home on Sunday, the 30th of October. Sandbrook came first: he came about three o'clock. It was near six o'clock when Grainger came. When Grainger came, he peeped round the screen, and then Sandbrook followed him into the parlour.

Sandbrook said, the parlour was cooler than the other room. They drank two jugs of ale, and remained together about half-an-hour.

Cross-examined.—My house is a public house. There were many other customers in the house at the time Grainger and Sandbrook were there.

Re-examined.— Grainger and Sandbrook were talking and drinking together.

Mr. Whateley said that was the case on the part of the prosecution.

Mr. CORBETT then addressed the Jury, on the part of Grainger. At the outset, he besought the Jury to divest their minds of all prejudice, respecting the nature of the charge against the prisoner for whom he appeared,— an offence which, he knew, was peculiarly odious in the eyes of the public; and to confine their attention to the evidence brought against him. He was sure, if they succeeded in doing so, they must come to the conclusion that there was not the slightest evidence to warrant their finding a verdict of guilty against Grainger. The learned Counsel then contended that the fact of Grainger being seen in the company of Sandbrook on the day before the offence was committed was an occurrence which might have happened to any person, and that no proof of guilt could be gathered from it; and ingeniously argued that Grainger's motive for denying any knowledge of Sandbrook might arise from a desire to be considered altogether unconnected with a person charged with an offence which had excited so much popular hatred. The Learned Counsel also maintained, that even if Grainger had a knowledge of the transaction in which Sandbrook had engaged, still he did not thereby make himself a guilty participator in the crime. He denied, however, that there was any evidence of Grainger possessing such a knowledge. The circumstance of the dirty coat did not call for a single remark from him – it was utterly unworthy of notice. The Learned Counsel concluded by saying that, not notwithstanding the case had been exceedingly well "got up." And many trifling incidents raked together to support the charge against the prisoner Grainger, yet that no proof had been given of his being an active participator in the crime, and they would, therefore, do their duty by acquitting him. A paper was handed up to the Chairman by Sandbrook, which stated that he was asked by a person – [The Chairman did not disclose the name] – to wheel the barrow, and that he did not know what was in it.

A paper was handed up to the Chairman by Sandbrook, which stated that he was asked by a person – [The Chairman did not disclose the name] – to wheel the barrow, and that he did not know what was in it.

The CHAIRMAN, after summing up, observed that the evidence against Grainger was very slight; and that if the Jury entertained any doubt of his guilt, they must give him the benefit of that doubt, and acquit him.

The Jury, after consulting together for a short time, found a verict of guilty against both prisoners.

The CHAIRMAN then told Grainger that he had been tried before for a similar offence, and was known to be addicted to the practice of disinterring dead bodies.

He believed that Sandbrook had been a mere instrument in his hands; he should therefore pass a much more severe sentence upon him (Grainger) than upon Sandbrook. Grainger – to be imprisoned six months, to hard labour, and to pay a fine of 10/-. Sandbrook – to be imprisoned one month.

Before the prisoners quitted the bar, Grainger threw a written paper upon the barristers' table, which was addressed to the Chairman.

Sir O.MOSLEY, after reading it, called up Scott, the constable, and told him that the prisoners charged him with having placed them before a roasting fire, chained and kept them there for a long period, until blisters arose upon their hands & faces, in order to extort a confession.

Scott denied the charge altogether

The CHAIRMAN said it was a serious charge; and asked if he could disprove it.

Scott then called upon

W. Dibb, one of the officers of the County Prison, who said that upon the prisoners being brought to Stafford, they had no blisters nor marks of burning upon their hands and faces.

Charles Heamhurst, the constable of Harborne, also declared that he saw the prisoners when in Scott's custody, and that although they were placed in a room where there was a good fire, yet they had the liberty of sitting near to it or far from it, just as they chose; and that they made no complaint of being scorched by the fire; and further, that he never heard Scott attempt to extort a confession from them.

Mr. WHATELEY said he wished to say a word on this subject. He did not now speak in his professional capacity; but he had happened to know Scott all his life, and he believed there did not exist a more respectable man in his station in society. He was utterly incapable of the conduct imputed to him.

The Court appeared perfectly satisfied with these exculpatory declarations, and the constable, Scott, retired.

This time the senior staff of the Birmingham School of Medicine and Surgery pleaded for clemency for Grainger alone:

School of Medicine Birmingham
January 9th – 1832

My Lord,

We the undersigned lecturers of the Birmingham School of Medicine and Surgery beg leave most respectfully to submit to your Lordships consideration the case of J Grainger convicted at the Stafford Epiphany sessions 1832 for stealing the body of J Fenton from the churchyard of Smethwick in the County of Stafford. Your Lordship will perceive from the enclosed evidence taken at the trial, that no case was made out, but from the prejudice which exists in the County from the prisoner having formerly convicted and imprisoned for a similar offence and though contrary to the charge of the Chairman the verdict of guilty was returned when a sentence of 14 months imprisonment and a fine of ten pounds was recorded. The prisoner Sandbrook against whom the case was clearly proved received a sentence of one month imprisonment.

Under the present circumstances we most respectfully trust that your Lordship will be pleased to recommend to his majesty that the sentence with respect to Grainger be remitted.

We remain my Lord
Your Lordships most obedient humble servants.
Richd. Pearson M.D.
John Eccles M.D.
John Birt Davies M.D.
G.B. Knowles
John Ingleby
John Woolwich

stealing[69] and on one occasion escaping from Warwick gaol[70]:

APPREHENSION OF A RESURRECTIONIST

Yesterday morning, about five o'clock, an elm box, two feet six inches in length, one foot six in breadth, and 14 inches in depth, was brought to Mr. Packwood's coach-office, in High-street, in this City, [Coventry], to be forwarded to ——, in London. The weight and appearance of the box excited some suspicion in the mind of the bookkeeper, and he resolved on seeing its contents; the lid was accordingly raised, when, to his surprise, he found the body of a young female in a state of preservation. In expectation that some enquiries would be made in the course of the day, which might lead to the apprehension of the persons who left it, it was deemed advisable to keep the discovery secret, and at five o'clock in the evening, a low sized young man, having on a white fustian shooting jacket and dark trowsers [sic], called at the office, and asked the porter who received the box in the morning if it had been sent off? The porter informed him that it was sent, on which the resurrectionist asked him to go out and have a pint of ale. To this he willingly consented and told him if he would go into a public-house near the office he would follow him. The fellow unsuspectingly went to the public-house, where he was soon surprised by the appearance of the porter and Davis, a constable, who took him into custody; when brought to the Police Office, he stated his name to be John Watts, but declined giving any particular accounts of himself. He was remanded for further examination.[71]

The discovery of the dead body created some commotion:

---

[69] p.4. *Coventry Herald*, Friday 9th April 1830.
[70] p.4, *Coventry Herald*, Friday 9th April 1830.
[71] p.4, *Coventry Herald*, Friday 2nd April 1830.

STEALING A DEAD BODY

We last week stated that a man had been apprehended with a dead body in his possession. On Thursday night last, a view having been taken of the body at the Police Office, the Mayor ordered a coffin and flannel dress to be procured; this was done on the following morning, and the body was put into the coffin and removed to the watch-house. Shortly after its removal, the same day, Mr. Burdett, one of the churchwardens of Wolston, being in Coventry and on Business, heard that a disinterred body was lying in the watch house, and knowing that some persons had been lately buried in Wolston Church-yard, it occurred to him that the body might have been taken from thence;; he accordingly went to the watch-house to see the body, and immediately recognized it as that of an aged woman, named Mary Rainbow, a pauper, who had been interred in Wolston Church-yard a few days before. He then went to the Magistrates, and having so informed them, Mr. Carter, the Superintendent of the Police, was sent to the Rev. Mr. Roberts, to obtain his permission to have the grave opened in which Rainbow had been buried; with this request the Rev. Gentleman complied, and on opening the grave it appeared the body had been taken away, the flannel dress and cap of the deceased being left in the coffin. The grave in which a woman named Hewitt had been lately buried, was next opened and found to have been also robbed. There was no other grave disturbed. To supersede the necessity of an inquest on the body of Rainbow, the Churchwardens of Wolston, and the nurse who attended the deceased during her sickness, came to Coventry on Saturday, and having identified the body, it was taken to Wolston, and re-interred.[72]

Watts was taken to Warwick Gaol by police Superintendent

---

[72] p.4, *Coventry Herald*, Friday 9th April 1830.

Carter, and committed to trial at the next Warwick Assizes:

STEALING A BODY

John Watts was indicted for having stolen the body of Mary Rainbow from a grave in Wolston Church-yard.

Mr. Waddington detailed the case on the part of the Prosecution; Mr. Amos defended the Prisoner.

John Smith, a coach-maker in the employ of Mr. Amos Packwood, of Coventry, said the Prisoner came to him about five o'clock on the first of April, when he was at work with a box on his back, and enquired for a coach-office. The witness said they were not up at the office yet, and he helped the box off his back, and told the Prisoner he would take it to the office when it was open, which he did. The box was directed – Pilcher, 35, Dean-street, London. The Prisoner said the box was to go by the Tally-ho coach, at half-past eight. He assisted the book-keeper to open the box and it contained some hat, a gag, and the body of a woman. The Prisoner came to witness again in the afternoon, and asked him if the box had been sent; when he pointed him out to a police-officer, who took him into custody.

Elizabeth Tew and Jeremiah Burdett, farmer, of Wolston, identified the body.

The Prisoner said some man, whom he did not know, had given him sixpence to carry the box to the coach-office.

The Chairman observed to the Jury, it was their duty to enquire, first, whether the body found in the box was the body of Mary Rainbow, and then whether it had been traced to the possession of the Prisoner, so as to convince them that he had stolen it or had been concerned in stealing it.

The Jury found him guilty, and the Court sentenced him to be imprisoned for four calendar months[73].

---

[73] p.3, *Warwick and Warwickshire Advertiser*, Saturday 24th April 1830.

It is no surprise that both Watts and Grainger supplied the same London based medical man, Dr. Pilcher. However, the sentence failed to deter him. Once released, he soon returned to the trade in Staffordshire and Worcestershire:

ATROCIOUIS OUTRAGE.—TWENTY GUINEAS REWARD
Whereas, on Sunday night the 2nd, or early on Monday morning the 3rd day of January instant, some evil disposed Person or Persons entered into the Church-yard belonging to the Parish Church of BURSLEM, in the county of Stafford, and then and there opened several of the Graves, in which dead Bodies had been recently buried, disinterred one of the bodies, which was afterwards found inclosed [sic] in a sack in the Church-yard, and took another out of the Coffin, leaving it entirely exposed in the Grave.

Notice is hereby given, that the above Reward of Twenty Guineas, will be paid by the CHURCHWARDENS of the said Parish of Burslem to any Person or Persons who may give such information as shall lead to the discovery and conviction of the Offender or Offenders.

N.B.—Two Men, one taller than the other, were observed near another Grave partially disturbed, with a Lantern, who upon an alarm given, immediately fled, leaving behind them the following articles: viz.

A broad spade, maker's name "Bache"; one pair of grey worsted stockings; a plain kerchief; a small hammer; a rough flannel top coat, of small size, with a quantity of nails in the pocket; one sack and one wrapper.

In a field, a short distance from the Church-yard, were found two Deal Packing Cases, 29 by 16 inches in length and breadth; which have been since ascertained by the Maker, to be the same Boxes that were ordered at his Shop, in Newcastle-under-Lyme, on Saturday the 1st day of January instant, by two men, one of whom appeared to be about 32 years of Age, 5 feet 7 inches high, florid complexion, stout person, round face, with a large scar under the left eye, and dressed in a white barracan [Barragan] *jacket, red plush waist coat, corduroy breeches, blue stockings, laced-up boots, and a white carter's frock.*

The other was apparently about the same age, about 5 feet 6 inches high, slender person, thin face, sallow complexion, with several of his front teeth out, and wore a rough flannel topcoat.

Persons answering the above description, were seen in Burslem Church-yard, on Sunday 2nd instant, one of whom had on a top coat, similar in every respect to the one which has been found.

By order of the Churchwardens,
P.E. WEDGEWOOD,
Solicitor for the said Parish of Burslem.
Burslem, January 5th, 1831.[74]

RESURRECTIONISTS. - Some of these wretches have visited Hanley Castle [Worcestershire], *in this county. It appearing that the ground in the church-yard had been disturbed, some of the graves were examined on Saturday, when it was found that two bodies had been stolen.*[75]

The names of the deceased were: Mr. Colson who had died three weeks earlier, and Miss Smith "...*a young lady of fortune, who died of consumption a fortnight ago*"[76], however, some of the locals took matters into their own hands[77]:

RESURRECTIONISTS. - We mentioned in our last two bodies had been stolen from the church-yard at Hanley Castle, in this county. We are glad to say, that through the activity of Mr. Cale, of the Anchor Inn, Upton, they have been recovered. As soon as it was discovered that the graves had been robbed, the resident

---

[74] p.1, *Staffordshire Advertiser*, Saturday 8th January 1831.
[75] p.3, *Worcester Journal*, Thursday 27th January 1831.
[76] p.4, *Morning Herald*, Wednesday 26th January 1831.
[77] p.3, *Worcester Journal*, Thursday 3rd February 1831.

Magistrates set on foot an enquiry. It was found that, at an early hour on the 21st ult. Two packing cases had been taken by two men, strangers, to the house of Mr. Cale, where a booking-office is kept for the Worcester coaches. The men nailed on the cards of the address with the kitchen poker and left them to be sent on to London. They were directed to "Mr. Naylor, Mr. Holmes's, Old Fish-st. Doctors' Commons." As there could be no doubt that these cases contained the bodies, Mr. C. went to London, where he arrived on Monday. Having obtained the assistance of a police-officer, he went to St. Bartholomew's Hospital, but here the enquiries produced no satisfactory result. They next enquired at the Belle Sauvage Inn, where they found that one of the cases had been taken to the house in Doctors' Commons, but that the direction had been accidentally torn from the other, and it had been sent to the White Horse Cellar, Piccadilly. On applying at the house in Doctors' Commons, the case was readily surrendered by Mr. Holmes, (who is a surgeon,) to the officer, and it had not apparently been opened. With regard to the other, it was found at one of the police stations, to which it had been consigned by a gentleman of the navy, residing at Pimlico, it having been sent to his house from the White Horse Cellar by mistake, as part of his luggage! The parties subsequently went before Mr. Alderman Smith at Guildhall, who ordered the cases to be delivered to Mr. Cale, at the same time highly and justly complimented Mr. C. upon his activity and zeal. Mr. Cale had returned to Upton, and the bodies have been re-interred. – There is reason to suspect the churchyard in question was violated in a similar manner in the spring of last year, when the same two men, the perpetrators of the outrage upon this occasion, are known to have been in the neighbourhood and had two packing cases of the dimensions of those recovered, made in Upton. These men travel under the guise of dealers in hardware; they have a horse and cart with them, but it is stated they make it a rule never to put up at any house, in order the better to elude detection, but pass their nights in outbuildings and under hedges. A reward of £10 is offered for their apprehension.

The surgeon, Dr. John Pocock Holmes (1783-1858) was the inventor of craniotomy forceps used in gynaecology, and the future author of "*A Treatise on the Employment of Friction and Inhalation in Consumption, Asthma and Other Maladies*" (1837) (Bloor 2023). He was not happy at having his name mentioned in the *Morning Herald* (26th January 1831). He replied, defending his reputation, possibly hoping to avoid a similar fate to Dr Robert Knox[78]:

TO THE EDITOR OF THE MORNING HERALD

SIR.— I observed a statement in your paper of yesterday, concerning a dead body having been taken from my house. Now, although I consider it no disgrace to perform dissections, without which no man can become, or remain a good surgeon, I do not like to be accused unjustly. I do not carry on dissecting at my own house, as I have opportunities of performing the necessary operations at two very excellent Anatomical schools, and therefore I never purchase subjects. The body taken from my house had been sent by some impudent resurrectionist, who may have known me at the schools, and took the liberty of directing it to my house, to be left till called for, supposing, doubtless, some of his crew would fetch the box away, and that I should never know what it contained.—I am, Sir, your obedient servant,

2, Old Fish-street, Jan.28.

JOHN POCOCK HOLMES.

It was not long before Watts was apprehended, with some incriminating evidence on his person[79]:

BIRMINGHAM RESURRECTIONISTS.—On Thursday, the Police of this town received a bill from Burslem, in Staffordshire, stating the particulars of the disinterment of two bodies in the

---

[78] p.3, *Morning Herald*, Thursday 27th January 1831.
[79] p.3, *Birmingham Journal*, Saturday 29th January 1831.

church-yard of that town, one of which was safely taken away. Immediately on the receipt of the advertisement, Hall, the officer, from the description given apprehended a notorious body-snatcher named Watts, alias Pointon, who has already been several times convicted at Stafford and Warwick for this offence, and once condemned, and imprisoned two years for sheep-stealing. There is every reason to believe that he is one of the party concerned in the Burslem grave robberies. When apprehended, the following curious document, addressed to a surgeon of considerable standing in this town, by his son in London, was found in his pocket:

"Dear Father- It appears that the man Watts, and his partner here, made a sad mess with the last packages they have sent. This morning two constables from the country called on Mr. Holmes, the surgeon, to whom the parcels were directed, and saw there the first box, which they immediately recognised from the following circumstance. It appears that Watts and the other man went into the house of the constable of the country, and actually borrowed the man's poker to nail on the directions to the box, and thus they (the officers) learned where the parcel was going to. The next day it seems part of the coffin, and a crowbar, were found in the burying ground, and the grave was open. This, of course, led to a suspicion as to the contents of the box; and immediately the constable set off for London, and detected, as I have mentioned, the first box, which contained a young female subject. This they took away with them, and requested Mr. Holmes to be at Guildhall at twelve o'clock: he accordingly went and waited till twenty minutes past, when, as these officers did not make their appearance, he left, and has heard nothing more of the affair, it being now four o'clock. We have heard nothing of the second package, and it is probable it has been either stopped on the road, or at the office in London. Mr. Holmes is a man of a very strong mind; he does not care a farthing about this discovery, which is so far fortunate, but we must alter the direction :- for the future, tell the men to direct to Mr. Smith, at Mr. Saunder's,

18. Devonshire Buildings, Great Dover Road, London, - They must have managed most wretchedly to go to the constable's house, and to leave the grave open. They must keep out of the way, as the officer knows one of them, and will soon take him into custody. Which it is I do not know, but if they do not mind, they will get taken. I write in haste, therefore excuse this scrawl.

London, Jan.24,1831   Yours, ever, R.D.G."

Hall, in the course of this day, will convoy Watts before the magistrates at Burslem.

However, according to the *Worcester Herald* (p.3, Saturday 5th February 1831)*: Watts was first "...conveyed to Bilston, on suspicion of having been concerned in the disinterment of a corpse in the church-yard of the latter place, in the course of the previous week."*

"R.D.G." was Richard Dugard Grainger (1801–1865) (see page 42), an English surgeon, anatomist and physiologist, the son of the Birmingham Surgeon, Edward Grainger. He ran the private Webb Street anatomy school, Southwark, London, before joining St Thomas's Hospital, London, as a lecturer. Grainger was also the brother-in-law of George Pilcher, mentioned above, who also lectured on anatomy, physiology, and surgery at the Webb Street School (Dictionary of National Biography 1885).

Watts appeared before the magistrates at Trentham on 31st January[80]. He was identified by a joiner who had made two boxes for him, for the packing of bodies, and had made two for him on a

---

[80] p.4, *Staffordshire Advertiser*, Saturday 5th February 1831.

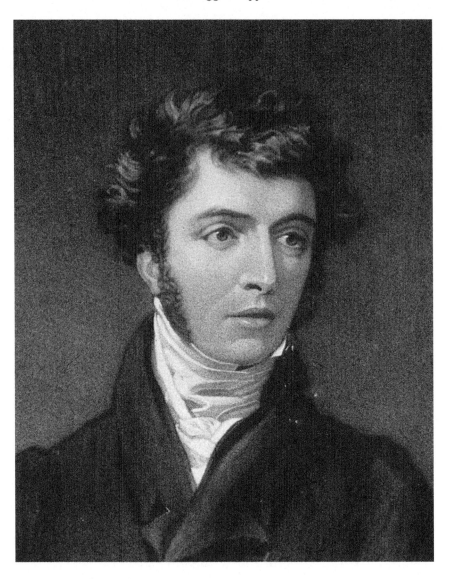

Richard Dugard Grainger. Mezzotint by T. Lupton (1827)
after T. Wageman.
(Wellcome Images)

prior occasion[81]. He was sentenced to twelve months imprisonment and fined £20 for the offence in Burslem[82]. The *Worcester Journal* (Thursday, 10th February 1831) hoped he would eventually be brought to Worcestershire to answer charges.

Watt's accomplice, George Riley, alias John Sharbrook, was also apprehended by Officer Hall, who arrested him while he was working at the Clay pits in Edgbaston. It was noted: "*Riley had been missing ever since the apprehension of Pointon*"[83]. Hall also conveyed him to Burslem:

RESURRECTIONIST.—[George Riley] *(28) was charged with breaking into a grave in the church-yard at Burslem, and taking away the body of John Goodwin, lately interred. Our readers will recollect that soon after the perpetration in January last, of the above offence, one man was tried and convicted of being concerned in it. His partner was the prisoner) ordered 3 boxes from him, which when made, they carried away in the direction of Burslem. A servant at the "Bull's Head," in Newcastle, deposed that on the same day, the prisoner and another man came to her master's house, and that they had a large piece of wrapping along with them. The sexton identified the defendant as a man whom he noticed peeping into the graves on Sunday the second of January, and whom he told to go about his business. This witness the next morning discovered that the body of John Goodwin had been removed from the grave during the night, and laid a short distance off, wrapped up in a cloth. A woman whose house overlooks the church-yard, deposed, that she saw two men digging there in the night, and laid a short distance off, wrapped up in a cloth. A woman whose house overlooks the church-yard deposed that she saw two men digging there in the*

---

[81] p.3, *Worcester Herald*, Saturday 12th February 1831.
[82] p.4, *Staffordshire Advertiser*, Saturday 12th March 1831.
[83] p.2, *Birmingham Journal*, Saturday 14th May 1831.

night, who fled on her making an alarm, and another witness picked up, within a few yards of the spot, the boxes which had been made by Lightwood. The prisoner endeavoured to defend himself by throwing the whole affair upon his companion, and declaring his utter ignorance of the purpose for which the boxes were ordered or used. He added, that he went to Birmingham, on the Sunday—Guilty. To be imprisoned for 6 months.[84]

In October, while still serving his sentence at Stafford, Watts died[85]:

DEATH OF WATTS, THE RESURRECTIONIST.—An inquest was held by Mr. Seckerson, in the county prison, on Monday morning, to enquire concerning the death of John Watts, alias Pointon, who expired on Sunday morning, in the hospital of the gaol, where he had been confined by illness since may last. Verdict, died by the visitation of God of pulmonary consumption. The deceased was under sentence of twelve months' imprisonment, for stealing from the church- yard of Burslem the corpse of a person of the name of Goodall, interred therein. Although a young man, (24), he was an old offender, having been imprisoned twelve months for felony in this gaol, and six months for stealing dead bodies before. Sentence of death was recorded against him at Warwick, where he suffered two years' imprisonment.

It is possible that both Grainger and Watts were members of the same resurrectionist gang.

---

[84] p.4, *Staffordshire Advertiser* Saturday 2nd July 1831.
[85] p.2, *Wolverhampton Chronicle*, Wednesday 12th October 1831.

3. STOPPING THE SNATCHERS

Attempts were made to deter the resurrectionists. Today several methods can still be seen in Scotland, although contraptions such at mort-safes would have been beyond the budget of most families. The most common method for the less wealthy would have been to keep watch over the fresh grave for two or three weeks until the body had decomposed sufficiently to be useless for dissection.

Watchmen were also employed to guard burial grounds and pitched battles occasionally took place between the guards and the resurrectionists, but some guards were open to bribery. *The Birmingham Journal* (Saturday, 4th November 1826) reported the case of Richard Dogget who was caught stealing two bodies from a graveyard:

The principal witness against Dogget was a watchman who seized him while dragging away a sack containing two corpses; but it appeared on the cross-examination of the watchman, that he himself connived at the practises of some resurrection men; from whom he received a sum of money for each body not to inform. A rival resurrectionist had offered a larger sum than Dogget, whose price was ten shillings to the watchman for each body, and the guardian of the night not finding Dogget willing to give more, took him up. (p.1)

When established in 1823, the Bilston Wesleyan Methodist Church graveyard had its own guard to watch over it:

... it was deemed wise to make a special provision for the protection of the graveyard. Andrew Allen, the caretaker, was employed to watch it, and was furnished with a gun, but was cautioned not to fire, should intruders come, until he had said three times: 'I'm going to shoot'.

This led to a curious incident. The Trustees had held a prolonged meeting, and had been quite forgotten by Andrew, who had retired to rest for the night, having carefully fastened the gates. When ready to leave they tried them, and in doing so made some little noise which was quite enough to rouse watchful Andrew. To their surprise his bedroom window casement flew open, and out came his head and gun, and instantly in rapid and angry tones he shouted: 'I'm going to shoot'. The dignified elders found cover with unusually quick movements, and shouted a quiet reassurance to Andrew.

Andrew had nerves of steel, a quick, salty wit, and a whimsical way of his own, and we cannot forbear another story about him as the graveyard watchman.

From the window of the old vestry he kept a keen eye on the burial ground, or sat in the late and early hours on a grave, with his heavy stick near, and his gun across his knee. This custom became known in the town, and some revelers at a Swan Bank tavern resolved to frighten him. For a wager one of them borrowed a white sheet from the landlady and started forth to play the ghost. Appearing at midnight, he remained quiet until St Leonard's chimes were heard marking the hour, when he walked towards Andrew, raising an unearthly moan as he went. Andrew sat quite still as the ghost drew near; presently he stealthily laid aside his gun and reached for his stick, saying: 'I shanna waste powder on ghoses – I'll try the stick,' and before the intruder was aware of his movements he was soundly rapping his head and shoulders with his cudgel, and had snatched off the sheet and torn it into many pieces, saying: 'I'll gie thee playing ghoses on me.' (p.137-8, Freeman 1923).

A similar incident occurred in St. Phillip's graveyard, Birmingham, in April 1830 when a grieving mother been standing guard at night over the grave of her infant[86]:

---

[86] p.3, *Birmingham Journal*, Saturday, 8th May 1830.

A GHOST LAID—During the last fortnight or three weeks, a woman named Marshall, together with a few friends, have been nightly accustomed to watch the grave of an infant, buried in St. Philip's churchyard, in order to secure it from the fangs of the resurrectionists. On Monday night, some mischievous wags in the neighbourhood, determined upon alarming this vigilant female guard; one of the party stripped to his shirt, and habited in a white night cap, made a sudden dart to the spot where they were assembled. All fled, save the mother, who immediately seized hold of the ghost by the skirts of his inner garment, and, notwithstanding his threats and imprecations, held him secure until she obtained the assistance of a watchman. He was immediately conveyed to prison, and on Thursday last, brought before the magistrates at the Public Office. The complainant not appearing, the prisoner was discharged.

At Alvechurch, Worcestershire, Billy Bourne, who lived in the church tower, guarded the churchyard armed with a sword and pistol until the mid-nineteenth century (Palmer 2005).

In Scotland, mort houses were also used, in which corpses were placed until they had decomposed and were then buried.

Booby traps were also utilised. One grieving father filled his child's coffin with gunpowder and fused it so that it would explode if disturbed. Another booby trap was the cemetery gun. These guns were set up at the foot of a grave, with three tripwires strung in an arc around its position. Those who stumbled upon one in the dark may have found themselves in a grave of their own, or seriously wounded. They were outlawed in 1827, (Guttmacher 1935; Orly 1999).

Others sought to make the graves of their loved ones secure against the resurrectionists by using coffins made of iron or mort safes, such as the one found at West Bromwich. The mort safe was

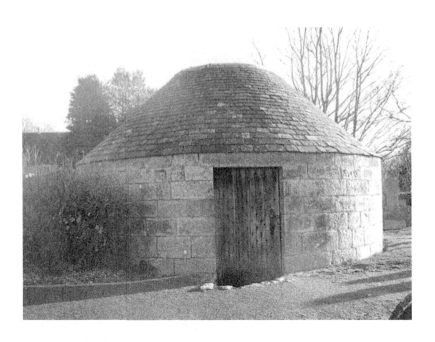

Nineteenth century mort house at Udny Green, Aberdeenshire.
(Photograph: Author)

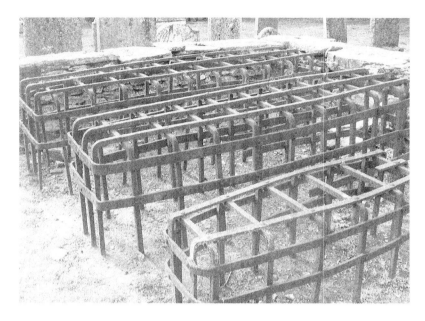

Mort safes at a church yard in Logierait, Perthshire, Scotland.
(Photograph Judy Wilson)

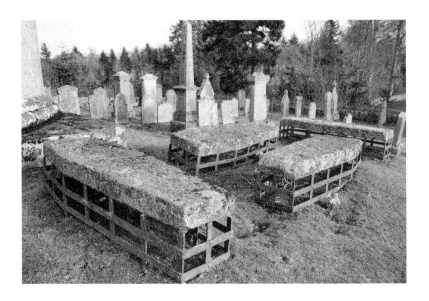

Mort safes in Cluny Kirkyard, Scotland
(Photograph Martyn Gorman)

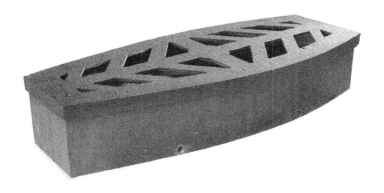

Iron Mort safe used to contain a coffin.
(Science Museum, London)

invented around 1816. These were iron or iron and stone devices of great weight, in different designs. Often, they were complex, heavy contraptions of rods and plates, padlocked together. A plate was placed over the coffin and rods with heads were pushed through holes in it. These rods were kept in place by locking a second plate over the first to form extremely heavy protection. It could only be removed by two people with keys. The safes were placed over the coffins for about six weeks, then removed for further use when the body inside was sufficiently decomposed. Sometimes a church bought them and hired them out. Societies were also formed to purchase them and control their use, with annual membership fees, and charges made to non-members (Lennox 2016)

The Birmingham Journal (Saturday 13th August 1825) carried a description:

SAFE BURYING.− The fulcrum, the wedge, and the pulley, have been often applied by resurrection-men to the exhumation of dead bodies, and too often have those mechanical powers drawn out of the grave the last remains of mortality. In order to disappoint the operatives who so dexterously remove the dead for anatomical purposes, a grave-digger, not destitute of mathematical knowledge, has lately invented an extraordinary interment, When the grave is dug to the depth required a cube of earth is taken out of the bottom, sufficient to admit the head of the coffin to be pushed half way in. Two stakes are then driven on each side of the coffin, and an iron is run through the stakes over the lid, so as to render the machinery used by the exhumators useless. The coffin cannot be removed and the dead may rest undisturbed. This mode of interment is now partially adopted.(p.4)

Other examples of attempts to deter the resurrectionists found in the West Bromwich Providence chapel graveyard included: a brick grave in which a corpse had been buried in two coffins - the outer coffin secured with thick timber and iron; a thick pine plank,

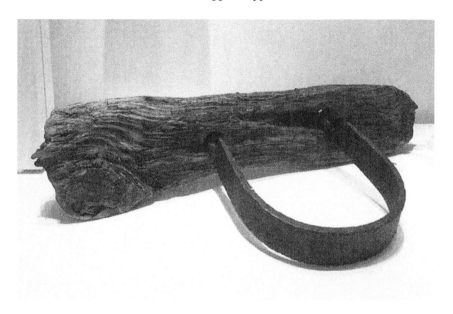

Coffin Collar: used to prevent resurrectionists stealing corpses.
It was fixed round the neck of a corpse and bolted to the bottom of the
coffin.
National Museum of Scotland
(Picture by Author)

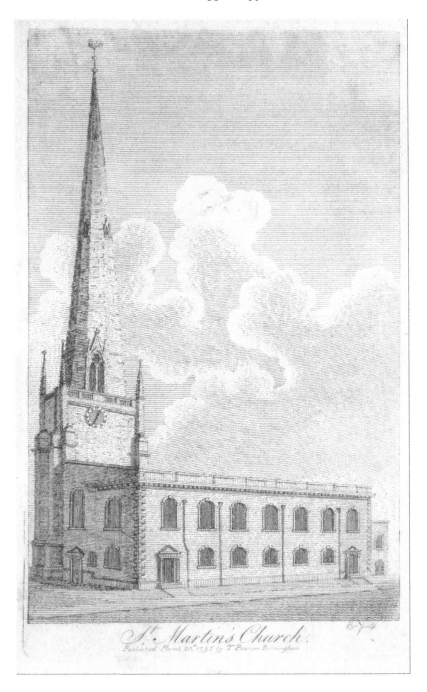

St. Martin's Church, Birmingham (1809)
From William Hutton *"A History of Birmingham"*

longer than the coffin, placed on top of a coffin and the ends recessed into the ends of the grave and iron bars laid across a coffin at chest and knee level. (Craddock-Bennett 2013).

The Staffordshire Advertiser (Saturday 7th February 1829) reported on the "*Schofield Safety Tomb*":

... a clergyman of the name of Scholfield has invented what he calls a "Safety Tomb," which will frustrate all the efforts of Resurrection men. From the last paragraph of the Rev. inventor's advertisement, it appears that the Safety Tomb will not only prevent resurrectionists from succeeding in their nefarious objects but will also punish them for the attempt. It says, "There are also such other contrivances within. (which it is not prudent to describe,) that if any person have the temerity to attempt an entrance after dark, or after the vault is secured, he must suffer the consequences of it." What those consequences will be does not appear,—we suppose they are too awful to be mentioned. (p.2).

Aris's Birmingham Gazette (p.3, Monday 9th February 1829) advertised extra secure coffins:

In consequence of the alarming reports that are in circulation in this town and its vicinity of bodies being stolen from Church and Chapel Yards, the Public are respectfully informed, that they may be supplied with WOODEN COFFINS, of which the maker will defy any possibility of their being re-opened by the Resurrection Men, at a trifling extra expense of a common coffin.

Apply to W. Faulconbridge and Co, Packing Box and Case-makers, Staniforth-street, near the Black Boy.(p.3)

Other methods included fixing a metal coffin collar around the neck of the corpse, thereby hindering the efforts of the resurrectionists. In St. Martin's churchyard and Park Street burial ground, Birmingham, brick lined vaults were also used as a deterrent

(Brickley et al 2006; Walker 2020).

Unfortunately, such protection was often only available to those who could afford it. However, other methods were suggested:

RESURRECTIONISTS. - A clergyman suggests the following plan, which he has adopted in his own church-yard, and has also recommended it to several of his friends: - Cover the coffin with earth, until within half a yard or more (as circumstances may admit), of the surface of the ground; then lower down the top stone which usually covers the grave, and afterwards let the whole be perfectly filled up, and remain so for about half a year or more, or if the friends of the deceased can afford it, a stone nearly the size of the grave may be gently let down into the grave, after each interment, having previously thrown about a half foot of earth over the coffin[87].

The *Birmingham Journal* (Saturday 16th February 1828) recommended another method:

HINTS TO RESURRECTIONISTS.— A plan has been recently adopted which appears likely to frustrate the exertions of the body snatchers. As the grave is filling up, occasional layers of straw or shavings are spread over the whole space of the opening, so that the insertion of a spade for the purpose of opening the grave is considerably checked, and the labour of the resurrectionist greatly augmented, if not rendered entirely abortive. When the grave of a female, in St. Martin's church-yard in this town, on Sunday afternoon last, this precaution was acted upon, and the novel spectacle presented itself of a man carrying a large bag of carpenter's shavings upon his back, as a necessary accompaniment to the funeral procession; this, no doubt, in accordance with the

---

[87] p.2, *Birmingham Journal*, Saturday, 28th March 1829.

request of the deceased, the calmness of whose last moments, probably, had been disturbed by the recollection of the late daring and successful attempts to supply the dissecting rooms of the anatomists.(p.3)

A similar technique was practiced at St. Paul's Churchyard, Birmingham in which long straw was placed in the grave, over the coffin, straw was then laid lengthwise, and sprinkled with earth, then more straw laid crosswise and covered with soil, and continued until the grave was filled with layers of straw and dirt, (McKenna 1992). While such techniques may have deterred the resurrectionists initially, they could dig a hole diagonally, exposing the end of the coffin, which could then be broken open and the body pulled out.

4. THE FALL OF THE RESURRECTIONISTS

In 1828 a governmental enquiry into the practice of anatomy schools made no specific recommendations into the activity of the resurrectionists and the medical schools, but strongly urged legislative action (Report from the Select Committee on Anatomy 1828). The Government was faced with increasing public outrage: over the Burke and Hare and *"London Burkers"* murders; the mass shipments of cadavers from abroad, and the fury of relatives having to protect the bodies of their deceased loved ones. An indication of the revulsion and anger felt by the public towards the medical profession were the Cholera Riots. In 1832, Britain was in the midst of a Cholera pandemic and areas of the West Midlands suffered severely (Goodman 2023). Riots broke out in Paisley, Scotland, and London over the suspicions that the corpses of cholera victims were being stolen by medical men for dissection[88]. On one occasion this was proved to be true: in Manchester, a boy who had died from Cholera was discovered to have been surgically decapitated. A riot ensued, and in the ensuing trial the magistrates concluded the head had been stolen for the purpose of dissection[89]. However, the West Midlands avoided such riots.

In 1832, the government halted the trade of the resurrectionists by introducing the Anatomy Act. Under the Act only licensed medical schools, physicians and surgeons had legal access to - i.e. they could legitimately purchase - corpses which were unclaimed after death in prisons, hospitals, asylums, and workhouses, providing no relatives of the deceased objected. It also appointed inspectors of places where dissections took place (the "Anatomy Inspectorate") and revoked the legislation permitting the dissection of murderers (Hurren 2011). The aim was to end

---

[88] p.2, *Staffordshire Advertiser*, Saturday 7th April 1832.
[89] p.4, *Aris's Birmingham Gazette*, Monday 10th September 1832.

bodysnatching and to protect the practice of anatomy by ensuring a lawful supply of corpses. This was something the medical establishment had long been calling for, including the doctors and surgeons of the Birmingham Medical School and the Worcester Medical and Surgical Society (Richardson 1988):

LETTER from Mr. Hodgson, Surgeon, Birmingham, dated May 6th, 1828, to the Right Honourable Robert Peel.

Birmingham, May 6th, 1828.

My Dear Sir,

I have received a letter from Dr. Somerville, requesting me to supply the Committee of the House of Commons appointed to investigate the difficulties of procuring subjects for dissection, through one of its Members, with any suggestions that have occurred to me as to the best mode of remedying those difficulties, as well as with certain information with regard to the state of Anatomical pursuits in this town, which induces me to take the liberty of troubling you with the following communication :

I am convinced that the feelings of the public can never be reconciled to the practices of dissection, so long as dissection continues to form part of the punishment for murder. The feeling, I really believe, in a great measure arises from the imputation which appears to be cast upon the character of the deceased, in consequence of his remains being subjected to that treatment which the law employs as a part of the punishment for the most heinous crime. I believe, therefore, that an alteration of the law on this subject is essential to reconcile the public to any facilities which may be afforded in procuring the only means of cultivating the most important of all the branches of medical and surgical knowledge.

Dissection being abolished as a part of the punishment for murder, I take the liberty of submitting to you the following, which, after much consideration, appears to me the mode by which the necessary supply of subjects for Anatomical purposes can be procured, with the least violation of private feelings. It is very similar to the plans pursued for the same purposes in some parts of the Continent; only I have avoided including the bodies of persons dying in prisons, because it appears to me very desirable to separate as much as possible the practice of dissection from punishment.

IT shall be lawful for the overseer of the poor, or his deputy, in any parish in Great Britain, to deliver to the surgeon of any public hospital or workhouse, or to any public teacher of Anatomy, requiring the same for the purposes of anatomical investigation, the dead body of any pauper who shall have died in the workhouse, or in any public hospital in his parish, which shall not have been claimed by any of the friends of the deceased, and which requires to be interred at the expense of the parish, under the following regulations:

1st.—The surgeon shall sign a bond, acknowledging the receipt of the dead body, and engaging to return the same within three weeks from the delivery thereof.

2dly.—The surgeon, on receiving the dead body, shall pay to the overseer, or his deputy, to be devoted to the funds of the parish.

3dly.—The overseer of the poor, or his deputy, shall, on the said dead body being returned, give to the surgeon a receipt for the same, and shall, within two days from the date ot the said receipt, cause the dead body to be interred in the same manner as if the said dead body had not been subjected to anatomical investigation.

4thly.—It shall not be lawful for the overseer of the poor, or his deputy, to deliver to any surgeon the dead body of any pauper as aforesaid, if it shall happen that the said pauper shall have expressed to the overseer, or his deputy, or in the presence of any two competent witnesses, his reluctance that his remains shall be employed as aforesaid.

5thly.—Any overseer of the poor, or his deputy, or any surgeon or teacher of Anatomy, who shall violate any of these regulations, shall be liable to a fine of to be recovered, upon oath, by an order from any of His Majesty's justices of the peace.

... I beg to state, that in Birmingham there are between

eighty and ninety medical practitioners, and about forty students. There is one anatomical lecturer, (Mr. Cox) who informs me that about twenty-five persons attended his lectures last winter, fourteen of whom were new pupils, the remainder were established practitioners, or non-professional attendants. The number of bodies dissected was eight. From inquiries that I have made, I have reason to believe that the workhouse in this town would afford more than four times that number of bodies, according to the plan that I have mentioned. Those employed last winter were, I believe, procured in the usual manner, by exhumation; and the discovery of this practice has caused considerable commotion and distress to the inhabitants of some of the neighbouring villages. Indeed, I am convinced that the occasional discovery of this practice causes far more annoyance to public feeling than could be produced by the adoption of a plan similar to that which I have detailed in the former part of this letter.

I have the honour to be, my dear Sir, your most obedient and faithful servant,

J. Hodgeson. (130-1, *Report from The Select Committee On Anatomy*)

However, the intentions of the medical men were less than altruistic. Thomas Wakely, the founder of the *Lancet*, observed that the purpose of the Act was not to ban the sale of cadavers, but to reduce their cost. Medical schools, and their governors, (a number of whom were members of the 1828 select committee which informed the 1832 Act, or providers of evidence to it), made a considerable amount of money selling parts of cadavers to students. While the Act covered the disposal of bodies, it did not include body parts or the selling of bodies and body parts. The resurrectionists had been setting ever-increasing prices for cadavers, and by flooding the market with bodies from poor houses and other institutions it was hoped the price would be forced down (Philip 2022). This situation had been satirized in the *Staffordshire Advertiser* (Saturday

9th November 1811):

Last week the whole of the corps, denominated Resurrection Men, employed in London and its environs, struck for an increase in wages! Last winter they entered into a similar conspiracy, and their anatomical friends acceded to the proposed advance of a guinea upon each body. At that time they received three guineas a corpse, and they now demand five guineas per body, male and female. The Surgeons have in vain remonstrated with them on the nature of their demand. They say they are fixed as death to their purpose, and many grave men among them raise up arguments in support of their extra claim. The matter remains unsettled. (p.3)

Some medical men did note the Act's exploitative nature, Dr. W.M.Horseley in *Cobbett's Weekly Political Register*, (Saturday 28th January 1832) observed:

The unfortunate persons who die in poor houses and hospitals have, in numerous cases seen better days, and have, during many years, contributed in direct payments towards the maintenance of the poor and the sick ... those of them who have not so contributed, have all been, so long as able to work, compelled to pay heavy taxes out of the fruits of their hard labour ... every working man ... pays full one-half of his wages in taxes; and that, therefore, when he becomes so poor, helpless and destitute, as to die in a poor house or in a hospital, it is unjust, cruel, barbarous to the last degree, to dispose of his body to be cut up like that of a murderer. (p.274)

The Anatomy Act was open to abuse. To Richardson (2001): *"What had for generations been a feared and hated punishment for murder became one for poverty."* (p.270-71). While relatives of the paupers who had died in such institutions could object to the bodies of their dear ones being dissected: they had to object within seven days of the death and provide the money to pay for a coffin and churchyard burial. If they couldn't afford this, the remains could - quite legitimately under the Anatomy Act - be sent to a teaching hospital for dissection in return for a fee which contributed to the income of the Workhouse. Some unscrupulous workhouse keepers posted notices of deaths in such convoluted language, only those who were competent readers would be able to understand their relative had died and be able to protest (Richardson 2001; Hurren 2011).

A debate in the House of Commons on 11th June 1844 confirmed that between 1839 and 1841, the bodies of approximately three hundred paupers had been dissected - quite legitimately - under the provisions of the Anatomy Act. It was also observed that not all workhouse masters were putting the fee paid for a corpse into the workhouse funds but were entering the death into the union's Dead-Book and then pocketing the fee for themselves. However, it was decided this was a matter for individual workhouse unions to address and not a suitable matter for Parliament to handle. It was also stated that when corpses and body parts were no longer required in one place, they were not being buried with the appropriate dignity and rites, but sold on, at a profit, to other hospitals and that lecturers were often adding to their own incomes through this practice. Once more Parliament refused to address the issue saying it was up to individual medical schools to control this. The plea of some Parliamentarians to set up a commission to investigate these matters fell upon deaf ears and their motion was soundly defeated (Hurren 2011).

Table 1 shows the number of bodies the Birmingham Medical schools received from 1833-1871. In 1849, Sands Cox wanted the inspectorate to persuade the local Workhouses to send all their unclaimed dead to his Medical School[90], a request which continued through the years, and resulted in disagreements with the

---

[90] National Archives Home Office Correspondence, Cox to Cursham, 1850, H045/3202.

Table1:
Number of bodies received at Birmingham Medical Schools from
1833-1871.
Compiled from Anatomy Inspector Returns
(National Archives: MH74/10)

Year	Number	Year	Number
1833	23	1853	20
1834	21	1854	7
1836	24	1855	25
1837	15	1856	26
1838	22	1857	27
1839	29	1858	15
1840	16	1859	21
1841	20	1860	16
1842	28	1861	16
1843	14	1862	20
1844	18	1863	16
1845	20	1864	15
1846	19	1865	19
1847	18	1866	17
1848	17	1867	22
1849	14	1868	15
1850	26	1869	30
1851	11	1870	21
1852	24	1871	13

rival Birmingham medical school, Sydenham College[91], over who should have the lion's share[92]. To Hutton (2016) Queen's College frequently received a very generous allowance compared with other schools nationally.

Some Workhouse Boards of Guardians refused to cooperate with the requests from the medical schools and the Inspectorate. In June 1838, the Aston Union guardians refused the request for bodies from the Queen's Hospital, Birmingham, *"taking into consideration the prejudice against and opposition to the Poor Law Anatomy Act."*[93]. In 1858, Dudley Board of Guardians also refused:

The Chairman laid before the Board a communication which he had received from Dr, Cursham[94], inspector of one of the schools of anatomy in London, stating that there was a deficiency of bodies for anatomical purposes, and inquiring of the Board if they would authorise the disposal of bodies of paupers over which they had jurisdiction. Owing to there now being two schools of anatomy in Birmingham,[7] the supply of subjects to that quarter was insufficient, and if the Board would agree to the request, the expense of the removal and burial would be born in all cases by the gentlemen connected with the schools of anatomy to which they were appropriated. Mr Darby said the medical gentlemen might perchance be sending the bodies back when they had done with them, and cause a deal of trouble. The Chairman of the Board

---

[91] The second medical school, Sydenham College was founded in 1851 as a medical school by a group of physicians and surgeons employed at Birmingham General Hospital at 12 St Paul's Square. It was named after the progressive English physician Dr Thomas Sydenham.

[92] For example, National Archives MH 74/10 December 29th, 1857.

[93] Aston Union Guardians' minutes Vol. 1, Birmingham Archives & Heritage Service, GP/AS/2/1/1, June 26, 1838.

[94] Dr. George Cursham (1795-1871): he had a modest practice in London and for some years acted as a physician to the Brompton Hospital, the Female Orphans' Asylum, and as a provincial inspector of anatomy schools.

advocated the surrender of all bodies in cases of suicide, believing that the instinctive dread which the people of this neighbourhood particularly had of being cut up, and examined after death, would be the means of deterring some people from committing the act of self-destruction. He, however, would oppose the giving up of bodies in case of accident or natural death. Mr. T. Griffiths thought the Board would not be paying due respect to the feelings of many of the poor if they suffered the bodies of persons under their care to be given up after death to the doctors. It was agreed that the Clerk should return a negative reply to the request.[95]

Queen's College approached Dudley once more in 1865 - despite having been warned by Dr. Cursham regarding their last attempt[96]:

A letter was read from the Medical Board of Queen's College, Birmingham, applying for bodies of deceased paupers for the purposes of the school of anatomy. The letter stated that the scarcity of bodies in Birmingham caused great inconvenience, as the students could not possibly receive proper instructions without cases upon which to operate. It also stated that the bodies were afterwards decently interred with full burial rites.[97]

The Board unanimously refused the request.

In 1873, the governors of the West Bromwich Union Workhouse declared that paupers in need of medical care had to come into the workhouse. However, if they died and could not afford a pauper funeral then their body would be treated as unclaimed and sold for a small fee to Queen's College Anatomical School in Birmingham. In this way their welfare debt to society would be

---

[95] p.3, *Wolverhampton Chronicle*, Wednesday 27 October 1858.
[96] National Archives MH 74/10 1st February 1865
[97] *Wolverhampton Chronicle and Staffordshire Advertiser*, Wednesday 15th February 1865 p7

repaid[98]. Mr. Hampton, a guardian of the Union, exposed the practice in *The Birmingham Daily Post* (p.7, 13th March 1877). At a meeting of the Union Board of Guardians, Mr. Hampton alleged, supported by Mr. Ward, (another guardian):

> *...bodies had been fetched away from the Workhouse by the kidnappers, body-snatchers, or whatever else they might be termed... the first body had been removed from that institution ... in a covered wagon by two men. The body was in a state of nudity, without any covering ... and its head was knocked about against one thing and another, thrown into the van, and treated altogether without respect.* (p.7)

Both men demanded to know how the bodies of paupers were being sent to the anatomy school, and exactly what burial rites were administered?

The Chairman of the Board and Mr. Gilpin, the workhouse master, denied the allegations. Gilpin responded:

> [A] *body to which* [they] *referred was properly dressed, put in a shroud and removed in a shell to the Dead-House. It was lifted into the coffin in the shroud, and was taken away to Birmingham in the coffin. He thought it was not necessary to have the body disturbed* [i.e. exhumed to ensure this was the case]. *He did not see the conveyance but was under the impression that it was a proper hearse* (p.7).

The Chairman emphasised that the journey of each pauper corpse from West Bromwich Union workhouse to the anatomy school at Birmingham was a *"Pauper funeral"*. It is interesting to note that the guardians did not refer to these procedures as *"Anatomy*

---

[98] p.4, *The Birmingham Daily Post*, Tuesday, 13th March 1877.

funerals". The latter title, while being far more accurate, would have caused outcry among the locals due to the stigma attached, especially as in a pauper funeral the body would be buried within the parish boundaries. The transportation of the corpses was done at night to avoid any bad publicity, but with the cat having been released from the bag, the Chairman was quick to reassure that the final burial of the remains was either in consecrated ground, if a Christian, or in a burial ground appropriate to the religious denomination to which the person belonged when alive (i.e. Roman Catholic, Methodist, Baptist, Quaker, etc.). However, he avoided giving details of where each corpse was buried, the state of the body when buried, and whether the body had been treated with dignity after dissection.

Union workhouse who supplied bodies to the Birmingham schools, including West Bromwich, Erdington, and Walsall[99], the Kings Norton guardians finally acceded to the Queen's Hospital in 1851[100]. However, the inspectorate was aware "*it could not fail to lead to some unpleasant consequences*"[101] when people discovered their recently deceased relatives were being sent to anatomy schools. This occurred on two occasions.

In early 1853, a body was taken from Wolverhampton Union to Queen's College School at Birmingham and the remains interred there. Shortly after, some relatives called at the Union and upon hearing what had taken place caused a great disturbance. The Poor Law Inspector intervened and the Board of Guardians was summoned. The resolution allowing bodies to be given to Queen's was at once resinded, and the supply from that Union was lost to the medical school[102]. Dr. Cursham "*... went down to W.hampton at the time (Feb. 1853) and saw the chairman of the Board, Rev.d Mr.*

---

[99] National Archives MH 74/10
[100] Kings Norton Union Guardians' minutes Vol. 5, Birmingham Archives & Heritage Service, GP/ KN/2/1/5, February 12th, 1851.
[101] National Archives MH 74/10 April 15th, 1861.
[102] National Archives MH 74/10 April 15th, 1861.

Owen[103], who was very anxious to serve the schools but a majority of the Guardians was averse, I suspect the Poor Law Inspector had to do with it"[104]

In the winter of 1889, James Clarke, a pauper, died in the Walsall Union Workhouse. The clerk of the workhouse noted that Clarke was a tramp with no relations and his corpse was sold to Queen's College, Birmingham. On the 10th December the Chair of Anatomy, Professor Bertram C.A.Windle[105], took delivery of it. The Anatomy Inspectorate was notified of the transfer. The body was released for complete dissection. Around January 11th, James Clarke's widow arrived at the workhouse. She was told by the workhouse master that her husband was dead, and the body had been removed. She left, completely satisfied, under the impression that her husband had received a pauper burial and been buried within the parish boundaries. On January 25th, Clarke's daughter, Mrs. Longmire, arrived at Walsall and made enquiries about where her father was buried. The Workhouse master informed Professor Windle who had the remains placed in a very basic coffin shell known as a *"deal box"* and buried on 31st January 1890 in common ground at Witton cemetery, Birmingham, in a multiple grave; the Rev. Thomas Rollison officiating. This ground had been allocated to the college by the City authorities for its own use.[106] The daughter's husband wrote to the master of the workhouse requesting information as to when the body was buried, and whether the whole of it was buried. Professor Windle also received a letter from Mrs.

---

[103] The Reverend Joseph Butterworth Owen (1809 - 1872)
[104] National Archives MH 74/10 January 6th, 1858
[105] Sir Bertram Coghill Alan Windle (1858 –1929) dean of the medical faculty of Queen's College, Birmingham and later professor of anatomy and anthropology and first Dean of the Medical Faculty at Birmingham University.
[106] National Archives MH 74/36 Letter to anatomy inspectorate 3rd February 1890.

Longmire on the 31st of January:

Sir,

On the 7th of December my father, James Clarke died in Walsall Union and his remains were forwarded to your college for anatomical Examination. I only learned last week of my fathers death and am grieve to hear from the Registrar of Witton Cemetery that other remains are buried in the same grave. As soon as I heard where my father was buried, I at once wrote for the ground to be reserved ith the sad result I have stated.

Will you kindly inform me whether there were any special circumstances in this case why my father's body was sent to you for such Anatomical Examination. I should also like to have a copy of your report on the case.

Yours faithfully,
M.A. Longmire
(nee Clarke)[107]

Windle replied:

Queen's College,
B'ham,
Feb 3rd 1890

Madam,

The body of James Clarke, so as you state forwarded to us for anatomical Examination.

The transfer was made to me under the customary regulations.

The certification of death states that death had resulted from bronchitis, and I saw no reason to differ from the diagnosis.

I regret that there should be any difficulty with regard to your father's grave. If I can be of any assistance to you in the matter, I shall be glad to help you. Kindly let me know whether you require

---

[107] National Archives MH 74/36 Letter to Prof. Bertram C.A. Windle, 31st January 1890

any further information and I will write to you again.

I am,

Yours faithfully,

Bertram A. Windle.[108]

On the same day he also wrote to John Birkett[109] of the Anatomy Inspectorate for guidance:

Their chief regret appears to be that they are unable to pitch a headstone as the grave is in common ground.

When they write to me again as they probably will do, I shall inform them of the fact, which they do not at present seem to have grasped, that their father's body has been submitted to complete dissection, and that the remaining fragments have been duly buried.

I presume that I shall be acting correctly in referring them for further information, as to the legality of the transfer and dissection to you?

I shall be obliged if you will inform me, if possible by return of post, as to whether I have acted correctly, and as to what further steps I shall take.

Am I right in concluding that the wife, and not the daughter is the first person who has a legal right to the body, and who therefore should complain in the first place?[110]

He replied:

Dear Sir,

I have carefully considered the subject of your letter of the

---

[108] National Archives MH 74/36 Letter to Mrs. Longmire 3rd February 1890.

[109] John Birkett (1815–1904) English surgeon and early specialist on breast disease, including breast cancer. He served as Inspector for the Home Office of the schools of Anatomy in the Provinces.

[110] National Archives MH 74/36 Letter to anatomy inspectorate 3rd February 1890.

3rd February and enclosed and I feel satisfied that you have fully carried out with regard to the body of J.C., removed to your school from the Wallsall [sic] W. house, all the provisions of the Anatomy Act relative to bodies consigned to Anatomy Schools.
Signed John Birkett[111]

In the file, housed in the National Archives, at Kew, London, just before the above correspondence is a copy of the Official Secrets Act with a handwritten date of 28th of November 1889. To Hurren (2011) this *"...has been pinned by a civil servant to the inside of the case file of James Clarke. It has been placed there to remind everyone connected to the Anatomy Inspectorate 'that the work of the Anatomy Department is covered by the Official Secrets Act 1889'* (p.70). The file contains a variety of documents from 1832 onwards, including letters, acts, and receipts. It has the appearance of being filed before the Clarke letters, rather than pinned as an imposing reminder.

While delivering presentations on the resurrectionists around the West Midlands, I have been told several times about occasions when elderly grandparents were being admitted to hospitals that were formerly workhouses[112]. They pleaded with their sons and daughters not to take them to the workhouses because they *"will cut me up when I die"*. It appears people were aware of what was happening.

---

[111] National Archives MH 74/36 Letter to anatomy inspectorate 5th February 1890

[112] For example, the now demolished Burton Road Hospital, Dudley was once the Dudley Union Workhouse; Gulson Road Hospital, Coventry, was Coventry Union Workhouse; Manor Hospital, Walsall, was Walsall Union Workhouse; New Cross Hospital, Wolverhampton, was Wolverhampton Union Workhouse; Wordsley Hospital, Stourbridge, was Stourbridge Workhouse.

Mere suspicion that a someone's body had been taken to be dissected was sufficient to provoke unrest:

ALLEGED NON-INTERMENT OF THE BODY OF A DECEASED PAUPER AT WOMBOURN

Within the past few weeks considerable uneasiness has pervaded the public mind at Wombourn, in consequence of the alleged non-interment of the body of a pauper, named Leming, better known, perhaps, by the soubriquet of Bolus – a title he had earned owing to an extraordinary propensity he was in the habit of exhibiting when tempted by offers of drink, for eating large quantities of food, swallowing candles, and other disagreeable commodities, Bolus, who, it seems, was formerly a corpulent man, had for some time previous to last Christmas suffered from consumption, and had been an in-patient of the South Staffordshire Hospital. Being considered incurable he was removed to the workhouse of his parish at Trysull, where he died in January. The funeral took place at Wombourn. Rumours subsequently gained currency that the body of the deceased was not interred with the coffin, but that it had been disposed of to a surgeon for the purpose of dissection. These rumours are said to have risen from a statement that the deceased while alive offered to sell his body after death to a medical man; that the master of the workhouse refused to allow the friends to have the dead body for internment, and that when the coffin was taken from the hearse at Wombourn churchyard it was too light to contain a man of the size and weight of the deceased. In this state of things the Rev. W. J. Heale, at the instigation of Leming's friends, wrote to the Secretary of State for the Home Department, asking him to direct an inquiry into the circumstances. The communication was handed to the Poor Law Board, by whose directions Mr. Kayne, one of their inspectors, attended at the workhouse at Trysull on Saturday last, and investigated the case. Several witnesses connected with the workhouse, together with some relatives of the deceased, were examined. The evidence of the former went clearly to prove that the body was buried in accordance with the usual rules. Two persons said they put it into the coffin; four persons saw it there, and two or more witnessed the screwing n of the lid, after which they said the coffin did not pass out of their keeping till it was deposited in the grave, nor was the body disturbed in their presence. It was stated that as the hearse approached the churchyard some friends of Leming met it, and wished to carry the coffin to the grave themselves, but this was refused in conformity with rule in such cases. The body, it was further explained, was much wasted by consumption, which accounted for the lightness of the coffin. Notwithstanding this evidence the deceased's friends present expressed themselves as not content, adding that nothing short of the opening of the grave and the coffin would satisfy them. The Poor Law Inspector said he should report the result of of his inquiry to the Commissioners. – [The coffin has since been disinterred and the body found undisturbed.][113]

A skeleton of a young male was uncovered, at the West Bromwich Providence Chapel that bore the signs of having undergone an autopsy: the skull had been sawn horizontally across the forehead and the vertebrae cut through, suggesting the spinal cord had been removed (Craddock-Bennett. 2013). Was this an autopsy? The remains of someone who died in a Birmingham hospital and whose body was claimed by his family for a private burial in their local churchyard, yet, unbeknownst to them, had been subject to dissection? Or someone who had been dissected in return for covering the cost of the funeral? Dissected skeletons have also been found during archaeological excavations at St. Martin's Church yard and Park St burial ground, Birmingham (Brickley et al 2006; Walker 2020), and Worcester Royal Infirmary (Western and Kausmally 2014).

---

[113] p.3, *Wolverhampton Chronicle*, Wednesday 5th June 1861.

Not all cadavers were transported to Queen's College in Birmingham. Professor Arthur Thompson purchased, on behalf of the Oxford University Anatomical School in 1886, two bodies from Wolverhampton Workhouse, and three from Birmingham; and in 1887 two from the Wolverhampton Workhouse paying £12 per body (Hurren 2011).

However, transporting the bodies via the stagecoach remained problematic, as the following incident in Birmingham illustrates:

DISCOVERY OF A HUMAN SKELETON AT A COACH OFFICE.— For some weeks past, the clerks and porters employed about the Castle coach-office, in High-street, in this town, were annoyed by strong and most disgusting effluvia, in an upper room, appropriated to the stowing away of unclaimed packages. As often, however, as the loathsome smell was complained of, no person, until Sunday last, was enabled to tell from whence it proceeded. On that day, however, upon proceeding to overhaul the boxes and parcels, it was shortly ascertained that the smell issued from a large deal box, which had been in the office for upwards of two years. Orders were immediately given to break open the package, and, upon the lid being removed, it was found to contain the skeleton of a human being! The box was immediately removed to the workhouse. An inquest was held on Monday evening, when it appeared from the evidence of Mr. Chapman, the coach proprietor, that the box came by a Liverpool coach two years ago, directed "to Mr. John Cohen, furnishing-ironmonger, Sackville-street, Birmingham," and that, being unable to find out any such person, or street, the package had been placed in the coach-office; but it was not until very lately that they had any reason to complain of the disgusting effluvia which led to the discovery of its contents. Mr. Cox, the surgeon, stated the skeleton to be that of a full-grown man, and it was doubled up in the box in the manner in which it was usual to pack subjects for dissection. The body was in a state of complete decomposition. The Jury returned a verdict of "Found Dead," but as regarded who the deceased was there was no evidence. There is reason to believe that the parcel was wrongly directed to Sackville-street, Birmingham, instead of Sackville-street, London.[114]

Did the Anatomy Act stop the work of the resurrectionists? Tales abound of the resurrectionists continuing their business after 1832. For example:

When Sydenham Medical College was located in St. Paul's Square, a well-to-do jeweler who lived a few doors down from it received a considerable shock one night. It was rather late, and he was getting ready for bed, when there was a knock at the door. On opening the door, a man standing there calmly informed him that he had brought the body. At the same time he tumbled a sack into his hall, much to the horror of the old gentleman. The man had delivered his "charge" to the wrong door. (p.18, McKenna 1992)

Soon after the opening of Queen's College, Paradise Street, in the mid-1840s, a senior student was left alone one Christmas Eve, to await the arrival of a body, which a man was to bring from Walsall. It was very late when he did arrive, and he was much the worse for drink. Instead of one body, he had two. All he could say about the second, was that he had found him. Nothing more could be got from him. (p.18, McKenna 1992)

About forty years ago, I was talking to a very old man who remembered as a child looking from an attic window in Icknield Street, Birmingham and watching lights in the Warstone Lane Church yard. His father told him, "The diggum uppers bin after Jobey Didlum". Jobey had been his playmate, recently dead. The medical school in Edmund Street a few hundred yards distant. (p.20-

---

[114] p.3, *London Courier and Evening Gazette*, Friday 27th January 1837.

21, Langley 1978)

To Palmer (2002) the body of Emma Foulger (14) who was accidentally shot dead by her brother Henry (12) in Aylton, near Ledbury, in 1855, was stolen from her grave.

One item that has been associated with resurrectionists is "The Hand of Glory" which was discovered in The White Hart Public House in Caldmore (pronounced "*Carma*"), Walsall. The building dates from the second half of the 17th century and was originally a private residence probably built by George Hawe. During the 1870's, while the inn was being renovated, workmen discovered a the arm of a child hidden in an attic chimney. It was originally thought to be a "*Hand of Glory*": a hand cut from a hanged felon, dried, and either by lighting the fingers, or using the hand as a candle holder, it would prevent the sleeping inhabitants of a house awaking while a burglar ransacked it. A pathologist's report in 1965 declared it to be the arm of an infant which had been skillfully dissected by a surgeon and injected with formalin to preserve it[115].

Formalin was not used as a preservative until the 1860's[116]. It may have belonged to a medical student, who fearful of the repercussions of being caught with such an item in his possession, decided to hide it, but was unable to retrieve it.

While such tales make for interesting local lore, apart from some sporadic incidents in 1833[117], reports in the newspapers soon disappeared, the trade in dead bodies had become legal and regulated. The resurrectionists were no more.

---

[115] The Hand of Glory: blackcountryhistory.org.

[116] Zhang, L. (2018) *Formaldehyde: Exposure, Toxicity and Health Effects*, The Royal Society of Chemistry.

[117] Rochdale: *Leeds Times*, Thursday 28th March 1833; Romford: *Essex Standard*, Saturday 28th September 1833

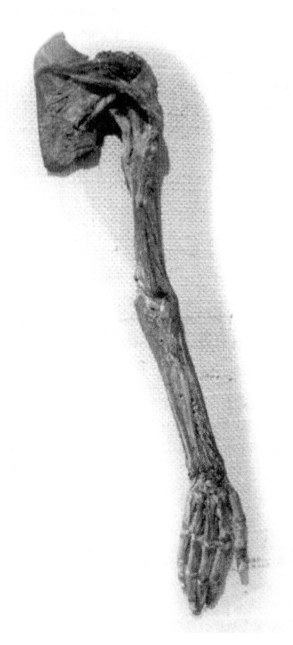

Hand of Glory from The White Hart, Caldmore Green, Walsall.
© Walsall Museums Service,

5. IT DOESN'T HAPPEN TODAY...

The 1832 Anatomy Act was not repealed until the introduction of the 1984 Anatomy Act which was introduced to address the issue of organ transplants. This was superseded by the Human Tissue Act 2004 (the Human Tissue Act, 2006, in Scotland) which made it illegal to remove, store or use human tissue without appropriate consent.

The Human Tissue Act arose from the scandals in the 1980's and 1990's at Alder Hey Children's Hospital, Liverpool, (HMSO 2001a) and Bristol Royal Infirmary (HMSO 2001b) in which both hospitals were found guilty of keeping organs from dead children without the consent of parents. However, in 2012 it was revealed that several police forces in the United Kingdom had stored the body parts of hundreds of murder victims without the knowledge of their relatives)[118].

Further, in 2015, it was revealed that the Biological Research Centre, Arizona, United States, which brokered the donation of human bodies for medical research had been selling the bodies to a United States Army research project for use in blast testing. The owner Stephen Gore was sentenced to between two and a half years to seven years in prison for mishandling the donations[119].

Between 2018 and 2023, human remains, donated for medical research, were stolen from Harvard Medical School's morgue, and sold by the former manager of the morgue. He would allow people to choose the body parts they want to buy at the morgue before taking them to his home and sending them from there (BBC 2023)[120].

---

[118] *The Guardian* 21st May 2012. *Police keep body parts unnecessarily.*

[119] *The Independent,* Wednesday 30 October 2019 *Body parts company secretly sold corpses for military explosives testing, court told.*

[120] BBC News. 14th June 2023, Harvard Morgue Manager Charged with selling body parts https://www.bbc.co.uk/news/world-us-canada-65910487.

APPENDIX 1

The Murder of Joseph Walker April 1759

Aris's Birmingham Gazette, Monday 16th April 1759, p3:

> *On Friday last a most cruel Murder was committed on the Body of John Walker, at Joseph Darby's near Hales Owen, where the Deceased and one Nathaniel Gower, as Bailiffs, were in Possession of the said Darby's Goods on a Distress for Rent: About Nine that Evening, the said Darby's two Sons, Joseph and Thomas, came into the House, and with a Broom-Hook and Bludgeon fell upon the said Bailiffs, and Gower escaping, they cut and beat the Deceased till he was almost killed; then stripping him naked, thrust him out of the House, and with a Waggon Whip cut him almost in Pieces: Gower made the best of his Way to Hales Owen, from whence some Persons went to the Deceased's Relief in a Close near the said House, who found him weltering in his Blood, and with great Difficulty carried him to Hales Owen, where he immediately expired. His Body now lies for an Inquest to be taken by the Coroner, a most shocking Spectacle to human Nature. Upon searching Darby's House early the next Morning, he, his Wife, and two Sons were secured, but not without great Danger to the Apprehenders, one of whom narrowly escaped being killed with an Ax with which the old man struck at him. They were all four Yesterday committed by the Rev. Mr Durant to Shrewsbury Gaol, upon full and sufficient Proof made of the Fact, and of old Darby's standing by, and all the Time encouraging his Sons in perpetrating this scene of horrid Villainy. The Deceased's Coat, Waistcoat, and Breeches, were at the Time of taking the Murderers found in the said House all bloody.*

Aris's Birmingham Gazette, Monday 23rd April 1759, p.3:

> *On Monday last the Coroner's Inquest sat on the Body of*

John Walker, who was murder'd by Joseph Darby and his two Sons near Hales Owen, and brought in their Verdict Wilful Murder. The Personwho first seiz'd the Murderers, and who very narrowly escaped being killed with an Ax by old Darby, was Mr Morson of the Town, who it is not doubted, will meet a Reward equal to his bold Behaviour on the Occasion.

Aris's Birmingham Gazette, Monday 30th April 1759, p.3.

To The PRINTER.

I Read with Pleasure, the Account in your last Paper of Mr. Mr Morson's being the immediate Instrument in apprehending the Darbies, for the shocking Murder of Mr. Walker: Indeed his Humanity to the Deceased in carrying him naked on his Back to hales Owen, covered with Blood, and mangled with eleven mortal Wounds, and his Care of him till he expired, cannot be too much commended; then his resolute but cool Courage, in seizing the Murderers, deserve the highest Applause. They were Fellows of the most daring, brutal Dispositions, who did not want savage Courage, and were become desperate by their Crimes: This was well known to Mr. Morson, and highly enhances his Merit in the Affair. But let us not omit doing Justice also to a Youth not more than seventeen, Mr. Wat. Woodcock, of Hales Owen, who alone, with equal Resolution, seized, and brought Prisoner to the Company, Joseph, the Younger and most desperate of Darby's Sons, as he was attempting to get off; while Mr. Morson, with the utmost Hazard of his Life, rushed into the House, and seized old Darby, his Wife, and the other Son. The young Men cannot be too much commended; sure I am they justly deserve the Thanks of the Publick. By inserting this in your Paper, I doubt not but you will oblige many, as well as Your and their (tho' entirely unknown)

Humble Servant.

Aris's Birmingham Gazette, Monday 13th August 1759, p3:

At Shrewsbury Assizes, which ended on Thursday, Joseph Darby and his two Sons, for the Murder of John Walker, in the Execution of his Office of a Bailiff, at their House near Hales Owen, were condemn'd, and on Saturday were executed. The two Sons are to be hung in Chains near Hales Owen, and the Old man's Body is given to the Surgeons for Dissection. The Wife of Joseph Darby, who was tried for being concern'd in the said Murder, was acquitted.

APPENDIX 2

Abel Hill

Staffordshire Advertiser, Saturday 25th March 1820, p.4:

A horrid murder, and of a peculiarly atrocious character, was perpetuated in the liberty of Bilston, about a month since; we belief on the 23rd ult. A woman named Mary Martin, and her infant natural child, were found in the Birmingham canal, near Bradley, with such evident marks of violence upon them as to leave no doubt of their having been wilfully murdered. The event naturally excited a strong sensation in the neighbourhood, and as several circumstances tended to criminate one Abel Hill, by whom the woman had the child, and by whom also she was again far advanced in pregnancy, he was apprehended and lodged in Wolverhampton house of correction. An inquest has been held at Bilston, upon the woman and child, and on Thursday the Coroner's Jury, after four days of most anxious and minute investigation, returned a verdict of wilful murder against Hill, who has accordingly been committed to our county gaol, to take his trial at the Summer Assizes.

Staffordshire Advertiser, Saturday 29th July 1820, p.4:

TRIAL AND
EXECUTION OF ABEL HILL
For the wilful murder of Mary Martin, and her infant Son, in the parish of Wolverhampton, and county of Stafford.

[Counsel for the prosecution: Messrs. Russell, Cross, and Powell – for the prisoner: Mr. Petit, Sir Wm. Owen, and Mr. Mac Mahon.]

Abel Hill was committed to our county gaol on the 15th day of March last, by Enoch Hand, gent. (coroner) charged with the wilful murder of Mary Martin, and her son Thomas Martin (a child about16 months old) by drowning them in the canal, near the Round-house, a little distance from Bilston, on the 23rd day of

February, 1820.

While he was in gaol, Hill appeared indifferent to his awful situation, and thoroughly disregarded religious instruction. Fully persuading himself that he should not be convicted, he sent to his parents with whom he had resided (at AbigaL Lane, in the parish of Sedgley) that he should be at home at the wakes. On the Friday preceding his trial, he was visited by a worthy Reverend Gentleman (who has taken great pains on similar occasions to bring sinners to repentance) who exhorted him to prepare for another world, as, in case of conviction, he would not be here after Thursday morning. Hill answered with a laugh, "I shall be somewhere else." In this hardened state he continued till the trial, which came on before Mr. Justice Richardson, on Tuesday morning last at eight o'clock, and was not finished until seven in the evening. It came out in evidence that Hill had cohabited with the unfortunate Mary Martin for more that six years, that he was the father of the infant child, Thomas Martin, and that its mother, the lamented victim of his brutality, was again pregnant by him. Mary Jeavons (the mother of Mary Martin by a former husband) was examined, and stated she kept a public house at Bradley, near Bilston; that the deceased would have been 23 years old on the 10th of March last; prisoner assisted in the support of her daughter's child, and seemed fond of it; her daughter and the child left her house about six in the evening of the 23rd of February last, and returned no more. Another witness proved that prisoner had endeavoured to cause abortion, by giving Mary Martin a powerful medicine, but it did not produce the intended effect. It also appeared that on the evening the murder was perpetuated, Hill had persuaded the unfortunate woman to meet him at Bilston, and bring the child with her, under pretence of purchasing it a hat and frock; and they were seen together by several persons in Bilston, and were also observed to approach the canal, as tho' on their way home. Cries of murder were heard from near the place where the bodies were afterwards found; the prisoner was also observed to have his shoes, stockings, and clothes wet a considerable way up his body, and marks of fingers and nails were found on various parts of the bodies, which proved that force had been used in drowning them. The bodies were found on the 3d of march by a boatman, the child about 40 yards from the mother. It was attempted to be shewn that the prisoner could not be the man who committed the murder, as he was at home at too early an hour to allow him time to return from Bilston; but unfortunately for the prisoner several of the witnesses for the prosecution proved his having desired them to mark the time when they saw him, on the evening of the 23d of February. One witness swore he had heard Mary Martin say she would make away with herself and child. The Learned Judge summed up in the most ample and perspicuous manner, commenting as he proceeded upon the nature of the evidence; and the Jury, after consulting about two minutes, returned a verdict of Guilty, which the prisoner heard without the least emotion or change of countenance. The Judge then passed sentence, in the most affecting and impressive manner:

Abel Hill, the circumstances of this most anxious and important case, in which you have been the principal actor, have engaged the attention of the Court a great many hours; more perhaps than was necessary to substantiate the case itself, but not more than was due for the satisfaction of the public. After a calm and dispassionate investigation, a Jury of your country have produced a verdict of guilty against you—a verdict which meets my entire approbation —looking as every English Court invariably does, simply to the evidence, without suffering the mind to be distracted by the tremendous circumstances of aggravation which have presented themselves throughout this most painful trial. You are convicted of the foul offence of Murder, not of one only, hardly can it be said of two—one almost your affianced wife, the object of your last and seduction, the other the offspring of your own loins, and probably a few months would have given birth to another. A case, I think, can scarcely be found, combining such a complication of terrible and appalling circumstances as yours. You appear to be a young active man, who was well and fully employed; led to the first commission of crime by your own lawless lust, and lastly to the perpetration of the present horrid business, by a mind callous to every feeling which should actuate a Christian, an Englishman, or any man; and sorry am I to observe that you are, perhaps, the most indifferent person present in this crowded Court. It is my duty to pronounce the sentence of the law upon you, which must be carried into execution speedily. You can expect no mercy here, for indeed mercy extended towards such a person as you, would be an act of the greatest injustice to the rest of mankind. You have a very short time, perhaps not 48 hours, to live, and let me entreat you to employ it well. For God's sake do not let your eye wander from object to object, but keep your attention fixed upon your awful situation. Do not imagine that by an apparent indifference and a denial of your guilt, you can extinguish the indignation of your Maker. The very short time which remains, for God's sake make the most of. Consider yourself as no longer a creature of this world, but endeavour to make your peace with the next; it is not too late to obtain the mercy of an all bounteous and all merciful God, if you set about it fervently, and employ day and night for its accomplishment. The sentence of the law is, that you, Abell Hill, be taken hence to the place from whence you came , from thence, on Thursday the 27th of July, to a place of execution, and that you be hung by the neck till you be dead; and that your body, when taken down, be dissected and anatomised; and may God, of his infinite mercy, have mercy upon your soul.

Whilst the Judge was passing sentence, the eyes of the prisoner were wandering round the Court, and he appeared indifferent, while the auditors were absorbed in grief. As he turned away from the box he exclaimed, "I wish I had a barrel of gunpowder under 'em, I would blow 'em all to hell."

After he had "returned to the place from whence he came," he made use of many horrid expressions, and although the chaplain attended him immediately, and continued with him an hour or more, he did not appear any ways composed, nor less violent against his prosecutors.

The Chaplain visited again on Wednesday morning, and continued with him upwards of eleven hours, using every possible means to tranquilize his mind, and prepare him for eternity; still he could not be prevailed upon to forgive his prosecutors. It being considered prudent to place a man with him in his cell, one who could read well was selected; but, though frequently urged, he did not once join in prayer during the night. He slept soundly from twelve till two, cried more than once at his untimely end, and about some young woman, supposed to be a sweetheart, but did not express any sorrow for the crime, which, indeed, he denied to the last moment of his existence.

On the morning of his execution (Thursday last) he was led to the chapel, where the sacrament was administered, and again the Chaplin used his best efforts to persuade him to die as a Christian, in charity with all men. The Reverend Gentleman succeeded so far, that the unhappy malefactor said he forgave every one. At five minutes before nine o'clock, he ascended the scaffold, quite undismayed, and making a spring up the steps. When the halter was placed round his neck, he desired to kneel, and did so, with the Chaplain; in this posture the rope became rather tight, and Hill said, somewhat jocosely, "It will throttle me." While the worthy clergyman read a prayer suitable for the occasion, Hill turned his head towards the spectators, and nodded to more than one, smiling at the time, and was totally regardless of the prayer. He soon sprung up with great agility, and the executioner having adjusted the halter, Hill pulled up his trousers, and skipping at the same time, shook off his shoes, saying, "I won't die with my shoes on; I'll make a liar of 'em." So anxious did he appear to look on the crowd, that he wanted the cap taken from his face, and the drop fell while he was asking to have it removed. He struggled much, but was dead in about two minutes. After hanging the usual time, his body was cut down, and delivered to Mr. Best, surgeon, who had it packed up and conveyed to Bilston, to be there dissected and anatomized, according to the sentence.

Hill was a very good-looking man, and well made, 23 years of age, about 5 feet 9 inches high, was born at Sedgley, and was employed as an engineer at the Deepfield Colliery, about half a mile from Bilston.

APPENDIX 3
Charles Wall

Worcester Herald, Saturday 5th June 1830, p.3:

> *Charles Wall, whose committal to our County Gaol, charged with the wilful murder of Sarah Chance, at Oldswinford, we stated in our last was asked in church to the mother of the child on the morning of the murder (Sunday). The act appears to have been committed with the most cold-blooded premeditation. Early in the morning, the prisoner enquired of a woman near the pits which of them had been "knocked off," meaning worked out; and shortly after nine o'clock in the evening, about which time it is supposed the atrocious deed was perpetrated, he was met in the ground in which the pit is situated, with the hapless child in his arms. She was crying bitterly for her supper, when Wall said, "don't make a noise, wench, I am going to get you some flowers." Shortly after, he was observed returning from the put without her. On leaving the inquest room to be brought to gaol, the prisoner said he supposed he should be hung.*

Worcester Herald, Saturday 31st July 1830, p.4 and p.2:

MURDER
> *CHARLES WALL, aged 23, was charged with the wilful murder of Sally Chance, in the Parish of Oldswinford, in this county.*
> *Mr. Whateley stated the case for the prosecution. The Learned Counsel begged to call the particular and patient attention of the Jury to the important charge he was about to bring under their consideration, as on their verdict depended the life of the prisoner. He them detailed the facts of the case, and called*
> *Mr. John Davis, who produced a map of the parish of Oldswinford, in which the pit where the body of the child was found is situate.*
> *Noah Stephens.– I am a miner; on the 19th of May I was at work in a lime-stone pit at Hay's Hill; I remember the signal being*

given for breakfast; it is by thumping the scaffold at the top of the pit; and when I heard the noise I ran from the breaks to the bottom of the shaft; I saw a bundle lying in the water; I thought it was my breakfast that had fell in; I got a stick and dragged it up, and saw it was a child; I was startled, and let it drop again into the water, and brought the child out; the water several days before was higher than on the day the child was found; the shaft of the pit was 240 feet deep; there are pieces of limestone sticking out of the sides of the shaft.

Cross-examined by Mr. Carrington.—Most of the children about that parish were dressed in check frocks.

W. Mudford confirmed the last witness's testimony.

Maria Pearson — I knew a little girl called Sally Chance; she was lost on the 16th May. I saw her in the evening, near the house of John Brooks; she was playing on the road-side with two other children. I know the prisoner; at this time he came up to the child and said, "Sally, your mother is gone home;" she said "Is her," and then walked away towards her mother's. The prisoner came out of Saml. Knowles's house; he followed the child; I never saw her alive again.

Mr. Davis stated, in answer to a question by Mr. Carrington, that there was no fence round the pits, and if the slide was withdrawn, a person might fall in by accident.

William Newey — I know the prisoner; I saw him about a quarter before nine on Sunday, the 16th of May; he was then near the Enville public-house. The deceased was walking about two yards before the prisoner; when I met him, he dropped down his head, and was walking with his hands in his pocket. About one o'clock in the morning he came to my house and knocked me up. I know the mother of the child; she came to my house about half-past nine to make enquiry after her; I said, "Mary, the last time I saw your child she was with Charles Wall." The prisoner was present, and she asked him if he had seen her; he said "he had not;" they then went away. The prisoner called me up at one o'clock, and said "Wm. Squirrel, (a nick-name) did you see me with the child?" I said yes;

he then called me a d—— liar. I saw the prisoner again about five o'clock; a man named Joseph Hunt was with him; he again asked me if I had seen him with the child, and on my saying yes, he again called me a liar.

Cross-examined—— I have often seen the prisoner with the child
before the 16th of May.

By the Judge — When the mother of the child made enquiry at my house, she was much distresses it was her lamentations that made me get up.

Mary Chance — I am the mother of the child; I live at the Lye waste; I am a single woman, and I know the prisoner. On the 16th of May I was at Samuel Knowle's house, from four o'clock to nine; the prisoner was with me; he left about twenty minutes before nine. My child was at the house about a quarter after eight o'clock; she asked me for a halfpenny, to buy apples, which I gave her; she then asked leave to go out to play; before she did so, she brought the apples to me; the prisoner was then present. Before I left Knowles's house, I went in search of the child, but could not find her; about half an hour afterwards I met the prisoner, and asked him if he had seen Sally; he said, "No, not since she brought you the apples." The prisoner went with me in search of the child until about o'clock, when he said he would go home and go to bed. I went to Newey's house; his wife told me that her husband saw Charles Wall take Sally Chance up the road; the prisoner was present and denied it. I had been at church that morning with the prisoner; he was courting me, and we were asked in church the first time that day. Wright Rubens was the father of the child. On the Sunday evening it was dressed in a light pinafore, and had no cap or bonnet on. I never saw the child again alive. I saw the prisoner next morning, and I asked him where the child was, and he said he did not know.

Cross-examined.— The prisoner used to call the child "Sally," I never knew him walk out with her before the day she was lost. I have another child about 3 years old.

By the Judge.– The prisoner did not help to maintain either of the children.

Thos. Kendrick.–I know the prisoner; saw him about a quarter before nine o'clock on Sunday, the 16th May. I know it was about this time, as I heard the clock shortly afterwards strike nine. He was near the Enville public-house; the roads divide at that place, and the prisoner was taking the one leading to the fields; the child was a few yards behind him; he called to her, and told her to come forwards; the child made haste, and ran after him; I then saw him get over the stile, but saw nothing of him again that night. About five o'clock the next morning, I went to the prisoner's house; he was in bed; I told him to get up; the constable was with me at this time: when he got up, I asked him if he had seen the child, and he said no, not since eight o'clock. We then took him to the pit, where we supposed the child was.

Cross-examined.– The stile where the prisoner got over with the child was not in the road leading to Mary Chance's house.

A prisoner named William Pritchard was the next witness called. The Surgeon of the gaol, however, stated the witness was quite deaf, and, in his opinion, insane; at times he was violent. Mr. Justice Park, in consequence, refused to receive his evidence.

William Baker– I live at Bretel-lane, near Oldswinford. I was at the Swan Inn, Lye Waste, on the 16th May. I left about ten minutes before nine o'clock; I went up the Birmingham road until I| got near the lime pits, when I met Charles wall; a young girl was with him; the child was in his arms; I did not know the prisoner before, but I am sure he was the man; I pointed him out at the inquest from amongst 13 or 14 people. When I met the child she was crying, and wanted to go home and get some victuals. He said: "don't cry, my child, and I will get you some flowers." I then bid him good night, but he did not answer. I got over the stile first, and the prisoner went towards the lime pits. I watched him down 30 or 40 yards; the child was still with him, and making a cry. I saw him within about 100 yards of the lime pits. I took particular notice of him, on account of the child crying so very much.

John Round.– I saw the prisoner a little after nine o'clock on the 16th of May; he was in the Hay's lane, between the stile leading to the pits and the Birmingham road; no one was with him at that time, I must have seen them if there had, as I passed close by him.

Jane Southall.– I live at the Hays; my husband is clerk to the owner of the lime pits; on Sunday morning, the 16th of May, about ten o'clock, the prisoner came to my house, and asked me if the road through a field leading to the coal pits was stopped; I said no, the road is not stopped, but the people are, as they do so much damage; he then asked me if I knew which of the pits was knocked off; I said that I had not heard my husband say a word about it; I then asked which he meant; he put up his hand and said, either that or that; I said, do you mean the lime quarry pits, and he answered yes; that was the one in which the child was afterwards found; no one was with the prisoner at the time he made these enquiries.

Cross-examined – It was well known in the neighbourhood that the pit was in full work, and had been for two tears.

Noah Stephens recalled— The pit was in full work at the time the body of the child was found.

John Yardley – I am the constable of Oldswinford I went to the prisoner's house on Monday morning to apprehend him; he was in bed; I told him the charge on which I took him into custody; he said he had not seen the child since a quarter after 8 o'clock. I then gave him into custody of Mr. Westward.

Wm. Westward.– After the coroner's inquest, the prisoner was in my custody; he said, "last Saturday I was very well off; I did not think it would have been in this way, I shall surely be hung for this crime." I said if you had not committed this depredation, you might have gone home with me.

Mr. Freer.– I am a surgeon at Stourbridge; on the 19th of May I examined the body of a child; the head was fractured; there was a very extensive lacerated wound on the scalp; it certainly was a wound such as might have been inflicted from the child being thrown down the lime pit, and was quite sufficient to cause instantaneous death.

This was the case for the prosecution.

The prisoner being called upon for his defence, said he left it for his Counsel.

Mr. Carrington, the prisoner's counsel, then called the following witnesses:—

Benj. Robins.— I am a nailor, and have known the prisoner 10 or 12 years. The prisoner always appeared to be very fond of Sally Chance; he was very kind to her and other children. I know the pit where the body was found; it is situated in a field where it is very common for children to play. I saw several children playing there about seven o'clock on the 16th of May; Sally Chance was amongst them.

Mr. Justice Park.— Take care, man, what you are saying; pray be careful.

Examination continued.— I brought one of my children home, and left the other playing near the pit. The prisoner was looking after the child on Sunday night. He was a very mild humane man, and was not in the habit of going to public-houses; he always bore a good character.

Cross-examined.— I saw the prisoner and Mary Chance about 6 o'clock; was smoking a pipe near the pit; Sally Chance stood by the side of me nearly the whole time; I left her there when I went away about 7 o'clock, with my eldest wench. I did not tell Yardley, the constable, that I saw the child playing round the pit. I told the child's mother of it about 10 o'clock on the same night. Charles Wall was with her; I said I have not seen Sally since I left her playing near the Lime Pits. I told a good many people of it; amongst others, I told Westward.

By the Judge.— I am sure I told the child's mother that I saw her playing near the pit.

Examination continued —I never told Yardley to keep the

prisoner in custody, as I was sure he murdered the child, and that I would pay all expences.

Josiah Hunt — I have known the prisoner 15 years; I knew the child from its infancy; the prisoner behaved more kind to her than I can do to mine; my children and others used often to play near the lime pits; I saw Sally Chance playing there on the 16th of May; the prisoner was a very honest and humane man.

John Cartwright (a boy ten years of age)— The prisoner is my uncle. I remember the night little Sally was lost; I saw my uncle on that night about nine o'clock at Hay's Hill; my brother and sister were with me; my uncle came up to us, and hid my brother Henry from me; he carried him in his arms down the lane; I afterwards saw my brother near the machine, my uncle having put him down.

Thomas Bolton – I live at the Lye waste; I have known the prisoner five years; his treatment towards the deceased child was very kind; he treated her better than I can do my children. It was very common for children to play near the lime pits.

Cross-examined.– I generally go to bed at 9 o'clock. I saw no other person in the lane besides Charles Wall; I don't know what Sunday night it was, but it was the same on which little Sally was lost.

Hannah Cartwright.–I recollect the night Sally Chance was lost; my children came home on that night between nine and ten o'clock.

Elizabeth Brettel.– I have known the prisoner for three or four years; he always bore a good character.

This closed the defence.

John Yardley re-called.–I know Benj. Robbins; I saw him whilst we were searching for the child; he told me to keep Charles Wall in custody, for he was the murderer of Mary Chance's child, and he would pay the expenses. He never told me any thing about seeing the child playing near the lime pits.

William Westward re-called.– I know Benjamin Robins; when I was searching for the child, he never told me that he saw it *playing near the lime-pits on Sunday evening.*

Mary Chance re-called.– I never walked with Charles Wall towards the lime-pits on the Sunday my child was lost; I knew Benjamin Robins; he never told me at ten o'clock on that night, or at any time afterwards, that he had seen her playing near the lime-pits. On being further questioned, the witness said, I was so distressed at the time, I cannot be sure, however, of what he did say.

Mr. Justice Park – You do quite right.

Mr. Justice Park minutely recapitulated the evidence. His lordship said he was at a loss to know what earthly motive the prisoner could have for committing so diabolical an act as the one imputed to him; but motives could not be judged by an earthly tribunal, they were open only to that Eye that knew all secrets, and from whom nothing was hidden. If they were convinced the prisoner threw the child down the pit, they must suppose it was from a malicious motive arising from some cause or other; and it would be their painful duty to find him guilty. But if on the other hand, they thought it fell in by accident, they would then return a verdict of acquittal. It had been proved by several respectable witnesses, that the prisoner was seen with the child going in the direction of the pit, about the time it was lost; it was also proved that he returned without it. His counsel had called witnesses to raise a presumption that the child might have fallen into the pit by accident.

Two witnesses were re-called, who stated that the mouth of the pit was invariably left open.

Mr. Justice Park — Gentlemen, on my summing up, I have all along presumed that the pit was left open, for had it been shut, it would only prove that the child had been thrown in by some wicked person or another, but it would not at all prove that the prisoner was the man.

The Jury then retired, and in about ten minutes returned into Court. The prisoner was then again placed at the bar, and the names of the Jury having been called over, the foreman pronounced their unanimous verdict to be GUILTY; and then addressing his Lordship, observed that it was the sincere and earnest wish of himself and fellow jurymen, that should there be, in his Lordship's judgement, any favourable circumstances in the case, that the prisoner should have the full benefit of them.

The most death-like silence at this moment reigned throughout the Court. The prisoner appeared unmoved, not a muscle of his face exhibited the least agitation, and he seemed stupidly indifferent to the awful situation in which he stood.

Mr. Justice Park — In a conviction for murder, Gentlemen, I can receive no recommendation for mercy; there can be no mercy in this world.

The Learned Judge then addressed the prisoner, expressing *his perfect acquiescence in the propriety of the verdict. The finger of Providence had pointed out his guilt as strongly as if the deed had been witnessed by human eyes. If the child had fallen into the pit by accident, her playfellows would have immediately given the alarm. It was, indeed, difficult to imagine his motive for such a crime as depriving an unoffending child of life; but God alone could know motives. His was a crime which admitted of no mercy. He had behaved most cruelly to the woman whom he was about to make his wife — he had behaved most cruelly to her innocent child. "I intreat you, therefore, (said the venerable Judge,) during the short time the law of England allows you to live, to spend it in prayer and supplication for mercy. You have committed a crime for which, in a few hours, you must be cut off from the land of the living. You have but a few hours to live: let me beg of you, when, to ask for mercy; be earnest in your entreaties, and you may yet find it. Knock with penitence at the gates of Heaven, and they may still be opened to you, for with God there is plenteous redemption. Crave after nothing but forgiveness of your sins, and may the God of all mercy grant you forgiveness, through the merits of his Son. It only now remains for me to pass upon you the dread sentence of the law, which is, that you may be taken to the place from whence you came, and on Friday next, the 30th of July, be taken to a place of execution, and there hung by the neck until you are dead; and that afterwards your body be given to the Surgeons for dissection, and may the Lord God of Mercy have mercy on your soul."*

The prisoner was then removed from the Bar; the only agitation that he had appeared to manifest was a slight quivering of the lip; he worked with a firm step.

Worcester Herald, Saturday 31st July 1830, p.3:

Wall underwent the dreadful penalty this evening, at six o'clock (to which hour the sentence was deferred owing to the election), upon the drop over the Lodge of the County Gaol, and his body was afterwards consigned to the Infirmary [Worcester] *for dissection.*

REFERENCES

Anonymous Ballard (c.1820) *Not A Trap Was Heard.* Printed by Jackson & Son, Printers, 21, Moor-street, Birmingham.

Anonymous (1832) *The History Of The London Burkers; Containing A Faithful And Authentic Account Of The Horrid Acts Of The Noted Resurrectionists, Bishop, Williams, May, &C., &C. And Their Trial And Condemnation At The Old Bailey, For The Wilful Murder Of Carlo Ferrari; With The Criminals' Confessions After Trial. Including Also The Life, Character, And Behaviour Of The Atrocious Eliza Ross, The Murderer Of Mrs. Walsh, &C., &C.* London: Printed For The Proprietors. Sold By T. Kelly, 17, Paternoster Row, And All Booksellers In The British Empire.

Bailey, J.B. (1896) *The Diary Of Resurrectionist 1811-1812 to which are added an account of the resurrection men in London and a short history of the passing of the anatomy act.* London: Swan Sonnenschein & Co

Bennett, R.E. (2017) A Fate Worse than Death? Dissection and the Criminal Corpse. In R.E.Bennett (ed.) *Capital Punishment and the Criminal Corpse in Scotland, 1740–1834.* Palgrave MacMillan.

Bhattarai L, K.C Sudikshya, Shrivastava AK, Sah RP. (2021) Importance of cadaveric dissection in learning anatomy for medical students. *Medphoenix; b6(2)*:68-72

Bolwell, J.S. (2022) *Surgery in London and the Royal College of Surgeons of England: Opportunities and Pitfalls.* Grosvenor House Publishing Limited

Burch, D. (2007). *Digging Up the Dead: Uncovering the Life and Times of an Extraordinary Surgeon.* Vintage.

Brickley, M; Buteux, S; Adams, J. and Cherrington, R. (2006) *St Martin's Uncovered: Investigations in the Churchyard of St. Martin's-in-the-Bull-Ring, Birmingham, 2001.* Oxbow Books

Craddock-Bennett, L. (2013), 'Providence Chapel and burial ground, Sandwell, West Bromwich', *Post- Medieval Archaeology. 47*:2, 382–6.

Dictionary of National Biography. London: Smith, Elder & Co. 1885– 1900.

Donnely. P. (2007) *Essex Murders.* Wharncliffe Books

Dudley-Edwards, O. (2014) *Burke and Hare.* Birlinn Ltd.

Frank, J.B. (1976) Body Snatching: A Grave Medical Problem. *The Yale Journal Of Biology And Medicine 49,* 399-410.

Freeman, J. (1931) *Black Country Stories and Sketches*: James Wilkes: Bilston.

Ghosh, S. K., and Kumar, A. (2021). Remembering William Hunter (1718-1783) the Pioneer in Obstetrics: A Prelude to Sestercentennial Anniversary of Anatomia uteri humani gravidi. *Journal of Obstetrics and Gynaecology of India, 71(1)*, 97–100.

Goodman, K. (2023) *"Nothing reigns here but Want and Disease, Death and Desolation!": The Black Country During The 1832 Cholera Pandemic.* Bows, Blades and Battles Press.

Goodman, N. (1944) "The Supply of Bodies for Dissection: A Historical Review". *The British Medical Journal.* 2 (4381): 807–11.

Guttmacher, A. F., *(1935)* Bootlegging bodies. A history of bodysnatching. *Bulletin of the Society of Medical History.* 4, 353-412.

Hackwood F.W. (1924) *Staffordshire Customs, Superstitions and Folklore.* E.P.Publishing: Yorkshire.

Her Majesty's Stationary Office (2001a) *The Royal Liverpool Children's Inquiry Report.*

-- -- (2001b) *The report of the public inquiry into children's heart surgery at the Bristol Royal Infirmary 1984-1995: learning from Bristol.*

Hurren, E. (2011) *Dying for Victorian Medicine: English Anatomy and its Trade in the Dead Poor, c.1834 – 1929 .* Palgrave MacMillan

Hutton, F. (2013) *The Study of Anatomy in Britain, 1700–1900.* Pickering and Chatto.

Jasper, J. (2014) Black Country Body Snatchers. *The Black Country Bugle*, June 18th.

Jordan, F.W. (1904) *Life of Joseph Jordan, surgeon: and an account of the rise and progress of medical schools in Manchester, with some particulars of the life of Dr. Edward Stephens.* London : Sherratt & Hughes.

Kirkpatrick, T. P. C. (1912) *History of the medical teaching in Trinity college, Dublin and of the School of physic in Ireland.* Dublin: Hanna and Neale

Lane, J. (2001) *A Social History of Medicine: Health, Healing and Disease in England, 1750-1950.* Routledge.

Langley, T. (1970) *The Tipton Slasher: his life and times.* Black Country Society

-- (1978) The Diggum Uppers in Jon Raven (ed.) Tales From Aynuk's Black Country. Wolverhampton: Broadside.

Lennox, S. (2016) *Bodysnatchers: Digging Up the Untold Stories of Britain's Resurrection Men.* Pen & Sword History.

London Medical Gazette: or, Journal of Practical Medicine. Vol. 3. London: Longman. 1829.

Lonsdale, H. (1870) *A Sketch of the Life and Writings of Robert Knox, the Anatomist.* London: Macmillan and Co.

McKenna, J (1992) *In the midst of life, a history of the burial grounds of Birmingham.* Birmingham Library Services.

McMenemey, W.H. (1959) *The Life and Times of Sir Charles Hastings.* London: E.&S. Livingstone Ltd.

Moore, W. *(2006) The Knife Man: Blood, Body-snatching and the Birth of Modern Surgery.* Bantam.

Morrison, J.T.J. (1926) *William Sands Cox and the Birmingham Medical School.* Birmingham: Cornish Brothers.

Nutton,V. (2004) *Ancient Medicine.* Routledge, London

O'Malley, C.D. (1964) *Andreas Vesalius of Brussels, 1515-64.* University of California Press.

Olry, R. (1999) Body Snatchers: the Hidden Side of the History of Anatomy. *J Int Soc Plastination 14 (2)*: 6-9,

Palmer, R. (2002) *Herefordshire Folklore*, Logaston Press..

Palmer, R. (2007) *The Folklore of the Black Country.* Logaston

Press.

Philp, J. (2022). Bodies and bureaucracy: The demise of the body snatchers in 19th century Britain. *The Anatomical Record*, *305(4)*, 827–837.

Porter, R. (1998) *The Greatest Benefit to Mankind: A Medical History of Humanity*. W. W. Norton & Co

Quigley, C. (2012) *Dissection on Display: Cadavers, Anatomists and Public Spectacle*. McFarland & Co

Reinarz, J. (2009) *Health care in Birmingham: the Birmingham teaching hospitals 1779-1939*. Woodbridge: The Boydell Press.

Richardson, R. (2001) *Death, dissection and the destitute*. London, Phoenix Press.

Rengachary, S.S., Colen, C., Dass, K., and Guthikonda, M. (2009). Development of anatomic science in the late Middle Ages: the roles played by Mondino de Liuzzi and Guido da Vigevano. *Neurosurgery, 65*:787–793.

Report From The Select Committee On Anatomy. Ordered, by The House of Commons, to be Printed, 22 July 1828.

Rosner, L. (2010) *The Anatomy Murders: Being the True and Spectacular History of Edinburgh's Notorious Burke and Hare and of the Man of Science Who Abetted Them in the Commission of Their Most Heinous Crimes*. University of Pennsylvania Press.

Walker, D. (2020) *Dissecting the past: Park Street studies shed light on how student anatomists honed their skills*. https://molaheadland.com.

Western A G and Kausmally T (2014) *Osteological analysis of human remains from the Worcester Royal Infirmary, Castle Street, Worcester*. Worcestershire County Council Archive and Archaeology Service

Whitfield, M. (2016) *The Dispensaries: Healthcare for the Poor Before the NHS*. Author House.

Wise, S (2004) *The Italian Boy: Murder and Grave-robbery in 1830s London*. Johnathon Cape Ltd.

Young, S. (1890) *Annals of the Barber Surgeons*. Appendix C.

London: Blades East & Blades, 1890.

About The Author

Kevin Goodman M.Sc., DHMSA, is a medical historian. He has appeared in several documentaries for television (including *"The Great Plague"* and *"The Black Death"* for Channel 5 and *"Mystic Britain"* for the Smithsonian Channel), and radio. He travels the country delivering presentations on the history of medicine and surgery to audiences in schools, museums, festivals of history and societies, and spends a lot of time being outwitted by his daughter.

His published works include:
Ouch! A History of Arrow Wound Treatment (2022)
The Lords of Dudley Castle and the Welsh Wars of Edward I (2014)
Quacks and Cures: Quack Doctors and Folk Healing of the Black Country (2017)
"Nothing reigns here but Want and Disease, Death and Desolation!": The Black Country During The 1832 Cholera Pandemic (2023)
Disease and Illness in The Black Country: A History: Medieval to Early Modern (2024)
All available from Amazon.co.uk

Buboes, Boils and Belly Aches: Essays on Health and Disease in the Black Country (2021)
Free to download from:
https://bowsbladesandbattles.tripod.com

More details regarding displays and presentations can be found at:
https://bowsbladesandbattles.tripod.com

Printed in Great Britain
by Amazon

45363937R00089